The Survival of Staff Development

Measure Outcomes and Demonstrate Value to Establish an Indispensable Department

Adrianne E. Avillion, DEd, RN

The Survival of Staff Development: Measure Outcomes and Demonstrate Value to Establish an Indispensable Department is published by HCPro, Inc.

Adrianne E. Avillion, DEd, RN, Author

Jaclyn Beck, Associate Editor

Elizabeth Petersen, Special Projects Editor

Emily Sheahan, Editorial Director

Adam Carroll, Proofreader

Mike Mirabello, Senior Graphic Artist

Matt Sharpe, Production Manager

Shane Katz, Art Director

Jean St. Pierre, Senior Director of Operations

Advice given is general. Readers should consult professional counsel for specific legal, ethical, or clinical questions. Arrangements can be made for quantity discounts. For more information, contact:

HCPro, Inc.

75 Sylvan Street, Suite A-101

Danvers, MA 01923

Telephone: 800/650-6787 or 781/639-1872

Fax: 800/639-8511

E-mail: *customerservice@hcpro.com*

Visit HCPro online at *www.hcpro.com* and *www.hcmarketplace.com*

Contents

Contents

Contents

About the Author

Adrianne E. Avillion, DEd, RN

Adrianne E. Avillion, DEd, RN, is the owner of Avillion's Curriculum Design in York, PA. She specializes in designing continuing education programs for healthcare professionals and freelance medical writing. She also offers consulting services in work redesign, quality improvement, and staff development.

She has published extensively, including serving as editor of the first and second editions of *The Core Curriculum for Staff Development.* Her most recent publications include *Learning Styles in Nursing Education: Integrating Teaching Strategies Into Staff Development,* the first and second editions of *A Practical Guide to Staff Development: Tools and Techniques for Effective Education,* and *Designing Nursing Orientation: Evidence-Based Strategies for Effective Programs,* all published by HCPro, Inc., in Danvers, MA, as well as *Nurse Entrepreneurship: The Art of Running Your Own Business,* available from Avillion's Curriculum Design.

She is a frequent presenter at conferences and conventions devoted to the specialty of continuing education and staff development.

Introduction

Survival in today's healthcare environment means that you must do more with less and do it efficiently. But it also means that you must produce quantifiable evidence to show that staff development is essential to your organization's continued existence.

The purpose of this book is to offer a survival guide for strengthening your staff development department despite the threat of downsizing and cutbacks.

It is your responsibility, no one else's, to prove your worth. It is my hope that this book will help you and your staff development colleagues develop a survivor mentality that enables you to:

- Demonstrate the value of what you do in a way that makes sense to colleagues from other departments and to administrators

- Evaluate your products and services

- Implement change based on evidence

- Offer cost-efficient, effective products and services that have a measurable impact on your organization

This material is designed to stimulate critical thinking about the process of staff development and to help readers thrive in a healthcare environment that demands objective evidence of how staff development contributes to an organization's success. No one person or department is guaranteed longevity in any healthcare organization. This book offers guidelines for strengthening your staff development department with evidence-based practices, aligning the staff development department's goals with organizational goals, and increasing your chances (and the chances of staff development) for survival.

Continuing Education Credits Available

Continuing education credits are available for this book for two years from date of purchase.

For more information about credits available, and to take the continuing education exam, please see the Nursing Education Instructional Guide found at the end of the book.

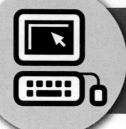

DOWNLOAD YOUR MATERIALS NOW

All of the tools and templates in this book are online for you to adapt and use at your facility. The files are available as Word® documents so they can be easily customized, and are organized to match the figure numbers in the book.

Find the materials by visiting the URL below.

www.hcpro.com/downloads/9561

Thank you for purchasing this product!

HCPro

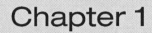

Chapter 1

The Realities of Staff Development: Survival

The Realities of Staff Development: Survival

LEARNING OBJECTIVES

After reading this chapter, you will be able to:

- Identify the characteristics of a survivor mentality

- Explain how to focus on evidence when analyzing staff development products and services

- Design a staff development departmental structure that facilitates the design and implementation of products and services

What Is a Survivor?

The definition of a survivor is one who remains alive or in existence. Additionally, to survive means (TheFreeDictionary.com, 2011):

- To outlive

- To persist

- To cope

- To remain

- To persevere (despite hardships)

All of these definitions are quite applicable to the survival of staff development, particularly "to persist" and "to persevere (despite hardships)." Persistence and perseverance characterize the nurses who helped make the specialty what it is today.

Staff development has evolved from what was once a 9-to-5, Monday-through-Friday job bestowed as a reward for nurses nearing retirement to a full-fledged nursing specialty essential not only to nursing, but to the entire healthcare organization (Avillion, 2008). Such an evolution would not have been possible without the efforts of nurses dedicated to the concept of lifelong learning that would ultimately have a positive impact on job performance and patient care outcomes.

Initial staff development efforts began with Florence Nightingale's work to establish training schools for nurses. Nightingale was a fierce advocate of lifelong learning. She was also one of the first to promote gathering data to determine best practices. Schools of nursing had strict disciplinary and performance requirements, and students, in large part, provided the nursing care delivered in hospitals. Much of the training was provided by charge nurses and physicians in the work setting. There was no true "staff development" department.

The majority of new nurses practiced independently, working as private duty nurses, often in patients' homes. However, the Great Depression of the 1920s and 1930s changed the focus of practice. Most patients could no longer afford the luxury of private nurses, and large numbers of nurses sought employment within the hospital setting. This shift in practice triggered the need for various types of education such as orientation, in-service programs, and continuing education. These endeavors were usually conducted by charge nurses, often as on-the-job training (Avillion, 2008).

Just as hospitals began to be the primary sources of employment for registered nurses, World War II changed the scope of practice yet again. Many nurses joined the armed forces, causing a significant shortage of active nurses on the home front. As a result, the number and types of nonprofessional staff increased, and nurses who had been inactive returned to work to help ease the shortage and support their families as spouses went to war. These changes further increased the need for orientation, in-service training, and continuing education, which in turn required more time and resources. The need for staff development nurses was becoming apparent (Avillion, 2008).

At some organizations, the provision of staff development services was not recognized as particularly important or arduous. Hence came the concept of "rewarding" long-time employees with what was viewed as an easy Monday-through-Friday job. However, those nurses (the original "survivors" of staff development) who recognized the link between education and job performance—and who were convinced of staff development's future as an important nursing specialty—began to evaluate the responsibilities and necessary qualifications for staff development specialists (Avillion, 2008).

This process of self-evaluation began in the 1940s and steadily progressed. In 1953, The Joint Commission for the Improvement of the Care of the Patient recommended that a department for the training and continuing education of nurses be established in hospitals. In 1969, the Medical College of Virginia's Health Sciences Division of Virginia Commonwealth University sponsored the first national conference in continuing education for nurses (Avillion, 2008; Tobin, Yoder, Hull, & Scott, 1974).

Today we reap the benefits afforded by those nurses who persevered in their quest to establish the specialty of staff development. Nurses can now earn specialty certification in nursing professional development (NPD), and resources specific to staff development are readily available, including journals, texts, and continuing education. We have our own professional association, the National Nursing Staff Development Organization (NNSDO), and, according to established criteria, we are expected to be prepared at a master's level of education (American Nurses Association [ANA]/ NNSDO, 2010). And yet, with all of the progress we have made, why is it that when budget cuts loom and downsizing becomes necessary, staff development is often the first department targeted for budget reductions and position eliminations? There is no simple answer to this question. However, it seems that we have failed, over time, to quantitatively demonstrate the impact our products and services have on job performance and patient outcomes.

We spend a great deal of time helping not only the nursing department, but, in many instances, the entire organization to enhance professional growth and development. We have helped implement evidence-based clinical practice, developed preceptor and orientation programs, facilitated research, and established career advancement programs for our clinical colleagues. We are critical to the success of achieving accreditation status such as that awarded by The Joint Commission and the ANCC Magnet Recognition Program®. But we have not taken the time to enhance the growth of our own specialty. Consider the following questions:

- Do you have a competency-based orientation program for staff development personnel?

- Do you have a career advancement program for staff development personnel?

- Is there a distinction among the levels of expertise of staff development personnel?

- Is the foundation of your department grounded in evidence-based practice (EBP) in staff development?

- Have you quantified staff development's impact on job performance and patient outcomes?

The answer to all of these questions needs to be "yes" if you and your colleagues are to be true survivors. It is important that we are as concerned with the growth and development of our own specialty as we are with nursing and the other departments we assist.

Characteristics of a Survivor Mentality

The survivor mentality is characterized by a combination of many things. Consider the following characteristics as you assess your own survivor mentality.

A survivor is never complacent

All too often we become complacent in our work. I can think of several colleagues who had worked diligently for many years in staff development in their respective organizations. They received excellent performance evaluations and were frequently assured by management and administration that staff development was a respected entity and not in danger of cutbacks. Nevertheless, all were affected by downsizing and budget cuts, and two were terminated in a major downsizing effort. As part of a noncomplacent mentality, you should ask yourself:

- Are you aware of the financial stability of your organization? Pay attention to any communications relating to cost expenditures. Read your local newspapers and visit your organization's websites frequently. Visit the websites of competing healthcare organizations as well. Sometimes local media representatives learn things about an organization's financial status that even managers and employees do not know. Is there any mention of pending legal action against your organization or its employees? Such action can significantly impact financial status. Never rely on one source for information about your organization's financial solvency.

- Are you aware of restructuring activities within your organization? Are certain departments losing positions? Are others gaining positions? Is there a pattern to the restructuring?

- Are you willing to ask managers and administrators the hard questions? Don't shirk from tough topics. Ask about budget cuts and budget projections. Discuss your concerns. Question how and why restructuring activities are taking place.

A survivor grounds staff development activities in evidence-based staff development practice

Create your staff development activities based on the following questions:

- Is evidence gathered for all staff development activities for the purpose of analyzing their impact on patient outcomes, job performance, and/or organizational effectiveness?

- Are all members of the department trained in the concept of EBP in staff development?

- Are staff development products and services developed and/or revised according to evidence?

- Are findings from analysis of evidence communicated effectively to other departments, managers, and administrators?

A survivor constantly pursues continuing education

Continuing your education is necessary in a world of rapidly changing technology and best practices. Studies suggest that there is a link between formal education and quality of patient care, so it is important to always be increasing your knowledge. When it comes to continuing education, ask yourself the following questions:

- Are you pursuing education in formal academic settings as well as via organizations/companies that offer accredited continuing education programs?

- Are you reading professional journals to help you remain current in trends in healthcare and staff development?

- Are you pursuing education that helps you identify potential positive and negative influences on healthcare? For example, are you pursuing knowledge of government rules and regulations that impact healthcare?

A survivor develops and maintains a strong professional network

Networking helps establish and preserve links between people who share common interests, so it is important for nurses to understand how networks are formed. Here are some ways to build new and existing relationships:

- Actively network within your organization. Make professional alliances among not only nursing, but other departments as well. If you can provide evidence that staff development activities impact the entire organization, you are more likely to enhance your credibility.

- Actively network with colleagues from outside your organization. Make contacts locally and globally.

- Become or stay active in your professional associations; these are excellent networking resources.

A survivor trusts her or his instincts

Develop and trust your instincts. If your instincts tell you that something is wrong, believe them. Then look for evidence to support what your instincts are telling you. For example, suppose administration assures you that there are no pending cuts in staff development. But when you talk to your manager, she is unable to make eye contact and changes the subject. You feel that trouble is coming. You have read in the financial section of your local newspaper that your organization is in financial difficulty. These factors should trigger anticipation of a potential downsizing. Make sure you have evidence that demonstrates staff development contributions to the organization!

> **STAFF DEVELOPMENT ALERT!** Even though you have sound evidence that staff development products and services have a positive impact on the organization, you are not immune to downsizing and cutbacks—no one is. But having such evidence and communicating it effectively will help, in many cases, impede these negative consequences.

Figure 1.1 offers a template for self-analysis regarding your own survival mentality.

The Survival of Staff Development

| Figure 1.1 | Analysis of my personal survival mentality |

Characteristic	Self-analysis
A survivor is never complacent	How do I remain alert to the organization's financial stability? How am I tracking restructuring activities in my organization? Am I asking the hard questions?
A survivor grounds staff development activities in evidence-based staff development practice	Am I gathering evidence for all staff development activities? Are all members of the staff development department trained in evidence-based practice in staff development? Are products and services developed and revised according to evidence? Are findings from analysis of evidence communicated effectively?
A survivor constantly pursues continuing education	In what settings am I pursuing continuing education? Am I reading professional journals? Am I alert to healthcare and staff development trends? Am I learning about government actions that impact healthcare?
A survivor develops and maintains a strong professional network	Have I networked with people from other departments in my organization? Am I networking with people outside my organization? Am I active in my professional associations?
A survivor trusts her or his instincts	Do I trust my instincts? Is there evidence to back up what my instincts tell me?

Focusing on Evidence

Being able to produce evidence that links staff development products and services to organizational effectiveness is imperative. This is the essence of EBP in staff development. It shifts the focus from what types of products and services we provide to how the products and services we provide impact patient care and job performance.

Ultimately, all staff development activities should be analyzed for a link between education and patient care outcomes and job performance. EBP in staff development is the foundation for this analysis, which involves the following actions (Avillion, 2007):

- Identify staff development products and services, beginning with those that have the greatest impact or potential impact on the organization (e.g., orientation, accreditation efforts)

- For each product or service, identify existing sources of data that will be translated into evidence (e.g., retention and turnover rates), how that data is collected, how often it is collected, and additional sources of data that could be used

- For each product or service, describe the mechanism for analyzing data, how often data analysis occurs, and how often products and services are reviewed and revised based on identified evidence

- Determine best practices and benchmarks for each product or service

- Verify conclusions by reviewing the literature and identifying current or planned research projects that will help further verify best practices and benchmarks

- Review and revise products and services based on the analysis of evidence in order to achieve best practices

Chapter 3 covers implementation of EBP in more detail. However, it is important in terms of survivorship that some points are emphasized here:

- **In EBP in staff development, all products and services should ultimately be evidence-based.** This means that data gathering is an ongoing process, as is analysis, review, and revision of activities. All staff development personnel should think in terms of evidence as they identify education needs and plan, implement, and evaluate education.

- **There is no such thing as "soft" data from "soft" programs.** In the not-so-distant past, some education offerings were characterized as soft, meaning their impact could not be measured. So called soft programs often dealt with emotional issues such as interpersonal communication skills or ethical issues. We now know that impact is measureable for all programs. If you are offering a communication skills program, it must mean that a need for enhanced communication was identified. Perhaps patient complaints regarding staff attitudes have increased or bullying among staff members has been reported and/or observed. The desired impact of a communications program would be to decrease complaints or bullying.

- **Staff development personnel should communicate using EBP as a foundation.** We waste countless hours in meetings trying to come to the point. By using EBP as a foundation, communication is clearer and quicker. For instance, when discussing nursing orientation with nurse managers, you need to speak in terms of how your orientation program is linked to retention data. If you need to speak to administration about the expense of a particular program, do so in terms of what evidence you have that the program is a benchmark for success. But be sure to relate what you mean by success. Explain how the program is linked to changes in job performance that have ultimately caused a decrease in infections, falls, or other adverse occurrences.

Survivors focus on evidence and how evidence is linked to a positive impact on organizational outcomes. Evidence gives you an objective focus that can be communicated in a clear and concise manner.

Staff Development Departmental Structure and Survivorship

The structure and reporting mechanism of your department is essential to survivorship. You must be seen as equal in status to other departments regarding not only structure and reporting mechanism but budget, staffing, and authority as well.

Staff development positions
Vice president of staff development

Large, multifacility health systems often have positions at the vice president level for nursing, therapies, information systems, etc. Positions in staff development are also beginning to be created at this level in such systems. An individual who has responsibility for staff development activities and all that they entail throughout the health system should have a title and financial compensation equal to those persons who also have multifacility responsibility. In other words, this position should be at the vice president level. Some organizations may try to design a position with the responsibility of a vice president but allocate the position to a lesser hierarchical level to try to save money. This indicates a lack of respect for what educators do and the impact education has on the organization. Beware of organizations that do not allocate staff development appropriately in the pecking order of an organization.

A person holding a vice president position in staff development should ideally be prepared at the doctoral level (ANA/NNSDO, 2010). This person will be responsible for the overall impact of education endeavors throughout the health system. Ideally, each facility within the system will have a staff development director who manages education activities for her or his facility and reports directly to the vice president for staff development.

However, vice president positions in staff development are still a rarity. Most staff development departments are still centrally located within one hospital or, at most, have responsibilities that cover about two separate facilities. Let's consider a departmental structure for these more common situations.

Professional development specialists

The staff development department generally has a manager who is a professional development specialist, prepared at the master's degree level (ANA/NNSDO, 2010). The manager's position should be at the same hierarchical level as other managers within the organization. For example, if your department is a division of the nursing department, the management position should be equal to that of the other nurse managers. If the staff development department delivers products and services to the entire organization, the management position should be equal to other managers (or directors).

> **STAFF DEVELOPMENT ALERT!** The hierarchical situation of the staff development department is important. It reflects administration's view of the importance of your department's products and services.

Nursing professional development (NPD) specialists and unit-based educators

The staff development department generally has a manager who is a NPD specialist, prepared at the master's degree level (ANA/NNSDO, 2010). Experience, expertise, and educational preparation vary depending on the role and responsibilities of the various members of the staff development department.

STAFF DEVELOPMENT ALERT! Make sure to differentiate between unit-based educators and NPD specialists. Survivors do not "lump" all positions into one category!

Remember that an NPD specialist has some experience in the field and is prepared at the master's level (ANA/NNSDO, 2010). A unit-based educator is an increasingly popular role within staff development. Prepared at the baccalaureate level, the persons holding these positions are generally responsible for in-service and just-in-time training, and helping the NPD specialist with more advanced tasks.

Survivors in staff development make sure that they work within a department that offers career advancement opportunities in the specialty. They need to know that there is a distinction among roles, and that as they acquire more skills and expertise, they will have opportunities to advance professionally and to be recognized for that expertise.

Figure 1.2 offers some recommendations for the identification of various levels of expertise in staff development and career advancement opportunities for each level. These levels are designed using Benner's (1984) levels of clinical nursing expertise as a foundation.

Departmental scope and reporting mechanisms

Departmental scope varies among organizations. The important thing to remember is that staff development must have equal footing with departments of the same scope and stature.

Housewide scope of responsibilities

In some organizations, staff development departments may have responsibility for providing services to multiple departments, sometimes even the entire hospital. If this is the case, the manager of staff development should have a title equal to those of others who have housewide responsibilities, such as the manager of therapies whose responsibilities include overseeing the delivery of therapeutic modalities, including physical, occupational, and speech therapies.

Reporting mechanisms should also be similar to others who have housewide responsibilities. For example, suppose those types of managers report directly to an administrator at the executive level. The staff development manager should also report directly to such an administrator. If the staff development manager reports to someone at a lower level of the hierarchy, this indicates that administration sees staff development as having lesser value than other entities with house- wide responsibilities. A survivor questions this and advocates for equal footing and equal respect.

Scope of responsibilities of the vice president

The role of the vice president is generally one that has overall responsibility for nursing staff development in a large, multifacility health system. In systems like these, there are generally a number of vice presidents who have multifacility responsibilities and who report directly to an assistant administrator or the administrator. If these positions are at the vice president level, it is imperative that the person responsible for staff development also hold the title of vice president and report to a similar executive-level position. If not, this is a blatant admission that education is not taken as seriously as it needs to be. This is a red flag. Staff development personnel should work long and hard to make sure this kind of inequality is corrected.

STAFF DEVELOPMENT ALERT! The best way to advocate for equal footing is to be able to provide ongoing evidence of the link between education and organizational effectiveness.

Nursing staff development responsibilities in a single facility

In single-facility organizations with a nursing staff development department, the manager of staff development holds responsibilities similar to nurse managers. Nurse managers are generally respon- sible for one or more units and report to the director of nursing or similar position at the executive level. The manager of staff development should also report to the director of nursing and hold a position of equal authority to nurse managers in the organization's hierarchy. She or he should not report to an assistant director of nursing or have a title of lesser value.

Some staff development departments allot responsibilities for identified units or departments (e.g., pediatrics or critical care) to specific educators. These unit-based educators should still report to the manager of staff development, not to the nurse managers of these areas. If staff development is fragmented by having educators report to others outside of the staff development department, staff development's scope of practice is diluted. Also, unit-based educators, in these cases, are often "pulled" from staff development responsibilities to fill in if the unit is short-staffed, help the nurse manager with managerial duties, etc. Staff development personnel should report directly to the person in charge of staff development!

In summary, a survivor is aware of his or her surroundings and what those surroundings say about the organization's view of staff development. This chapter offers suggestions on how to become a survivor or enhance your survivor mentality. Chapter 2 uses these suggestions to help you write a staff development business plan that enhances departmental credibility.

References

American Nurses Association and National Nursing Staff Development Organization. (2010). *Nursing Professional Development Scope and Standards of Practice*. Silver Spring, MD: Author.

Avillion, A.E. (2007). *Evidence-Based Staff Development: Strategies to Create, Measure, and Refine Your Program*. Marblehead, MA: HCPro.

Avillion, A.E. (2008). *A Practical Guide to Staff Development: Evidence-Based Tools and Techniques for Effective Education* (2nd ed.). Marblehead, MA: HCPro.

Benner, P. (1984). *From Novice to Expert: Excellence and Power in Clinical Nursing Practice*. Menlo Park, CA: Addison-Wesley Publishing Company.

TheFreeDictionary.com. (2011). *Survivor*. Retrieved March 30, 2011, from *www.thefreedictionary.com/survivor*.

Tobin, H., Yoder, P., Hull, P., & Scott, B. (1974). *The Process of Staff Development: Components for Change*. St. Louis: Mosby.

Writing a Business Plan That Helps Demonstrate Staff Development Value

CHAPTER 2

Writing a Business Plan That Helps Demonstrate Staff Development Value

After reading this chapter, you will be able to:

- Identify components of a staff development business plan

- Align the components of a staff development business plan with organizational goals and objectives

- Correlate the components of a staff development business plan with evidence-based practice in staff development

Introduction

Is a staff development business plan really necessary? Absolutely! A staff development business plan is not written merely to fulfill an organizational requirement. Nor is it a task to rush through and dismiss as a waste of time. A staff development business plan, written from the perspective of evidence-based practice (EBP), provides a guide for the development of products and services that have a positive impact on patient care and job performance. It should be a maximum of 15–20 pages. A well-written business plan needs minimal annual revision. Changes should reflect changes in the direction of the organization, updates to your action plan, and annual budgets.

Terminology may vary depending on your organization's philosophy. For example, the term "nursing professional development (NPD) specialist" may be substituted for "staff development specialist" depending on the structure and job descriptions of your organization. Likewise, the name of the department may be altered to reflect that of your organization.

All members of the staff development department must have input into the business plan. Because the plan provides direction for all staff development activities, everyone involved must agree with and support the plan. Ultimately, staff development personnel must design a plan that:

- Clearly supports organizational goals and objectives

- Correlates the components of the plan with EBP in staff development

- Provides direction for the achievement of staff development goals and objectives

There are a number of components that are common to most business plans, regardless of the business they drive. These are:

- Mission, vision, and values statements

- Departmental structure and description

- Products and services

- Marketing

- Action plan

- Budget

- Executive summary

Although the components may be the same, what makes a business plan really useful is to focus on writing a plan that provides the best direction for the achievement of necessary goals and objectives. Each section of your plan should have a good introductory paragraph. These paragraphs will ultimately be combined into the executive summary of your plan.

Mission, Vision, and Values Statements

Mission statement

A mission statement must clearly communicate the purpose and direction of staff development activities to persons within and outside the department. As with the vision and values statements, the staff development mission statement must reflect the content of the organization's mission statement (Avillion, 2008; Golway, 2009).

The sample staff development mission statement in Figure 2.1 describes essential functions as well as the overall reason for the department's existence.

Figure 2.1	

Sample mission statement

The staff development department of Major City Medical Center upholds the mission, vision, and values of the organization by planning, implementing, and evaluating education products and services designed to improve patient/family outcomes and the job performance of its employees.

The staff development department promotes the organization's goal of achieving accreditation as a leader in pediatric healthcare services. To facilitate achievement of that goal, continuing education programs that focus on pediatric healthcare services are offered not only to Major City Medical Center employees but to healthcare professionals in the tristate area.

The staff development department is committed to gathering and analyzing data for the purpose of identifying best practices and benchmarks in the staff development field. The staff development department is also committed to gathering evidence that links its education products and services to improved patient/family outcomes and job performance of its employees.

The staff development department shares its findings pertaining to best practices and benchmarks with the organization and with the community of staff development specialists via publication and presentation.

Vision statement

A vision is an image of what you want your department's future to be (Avillion, 2008). The staff development vision must coincide with the organization's vision. For example, suppose you have worked closely with the rehabilitation team whose members work to rehabilitate patients following stroke. You would like, as part of the staff development vision, to expand education in this field and achieve statewide recognition as a leader in stroke education. However, the organization's vision is to expand its pediatric services. This is a priority; stroke rehabilitation education is not. You must align your vision with the organization's vision and make pediatric continuing education (CE) a priority, as indicated in your organization's vision statement. To do otherwise is inviting conflict, and conflict can make the staff development department vulnerable to budget and personnel cuts.

A good vision statement is precise and easily understood by those within (and outside of) the staff development department. The vision should serve as a source of inspiration for all members of the staff development department and serve as a guide as you work together to build a common identity and future. In addition to inspiring, it must be realistic and obtainable. Such a vision is a source of pride and enthusiasm for members of the staff development department. An unrealistic vision, on the other hand, discourages more than it motivates (Avillion, 2008; Golway, 2009).

A well-written vision statement is (Avillion, 2008; Hiam, 2010):

- Clear

- Concise

- Driven by values

- Future-oriented

- Inspiring

- Realistic

Figure 2.2 is a sample vision statement appropriate for a staff development department whose organization is pursuing excellence in pediatric services.

Figure 2.2	Sample staff development vision statement

Major City Medical Center Staff Development Department

It is the vision of the staff development department of Major City Medical Center to be a tristate leader in the provision of continuing education that concentrates on pediatric healthcare services. These teaching/learning activities are designed to not only enhance patient/family outcomes but improve the job performance of those who participate in such education. Outcome data will be used to identify best practices in continuing education in pediatric healthcare services.

The vision statement in Figure 2.2 is written for a department within a medical center that has resources to achieve the rather lofty hopes it sets forth. It meets the criteria for a vision statement, but also reflects EBP in staff development. For instance, because the vision states that the teaching/learning activities are designed to enhance patient/family outcomes and improve job performance, staff development personnel must have a system in place to gather evidence to measure the impact of their education (see Chapter 3).

> **STAFF DEVELOPMENT ALERT!** Never put anything In your vision statement unless you are prepared to back it up with evidence of your accomplishments!

Values statement

A values statement, also referred to as a philosophy, describes the beliefs and principles that direct departmental activities (Avillion, 2008). Before writing a values statement for staff development, you must carefully review the organization's values statement. Your departmental values must reflect that of the organization.

Do the values of the organization reflect a commitment to ongoing CE and lifelong learning? If not, you need to approach management and administration and explain why such a commitment needs to be incorporated into organizational philosophy.

The values statement of staff development should contain references to the importance of lifelong learning and how teaching/learning activities are developed. It should also contain references to evidence-based staff development practice. Figure 2.3 is a sample staff development values statement.

Figure 2.3

Sample values statement

Manning and Wilson Health System Staff Development Department

Values statement

The primary responsibility of the staff development department of Manning and Wilson Health System, in collaboration with administration, management, and staff, is to plan, implement, and evaluate education programs that enhance employee job performance and contribute to desired patient outcomes. Education programs are developed and implemented within a framework of evidence-based staff development practice. Such practice is based on a continual analysis of staff development activities for the purpose of identifying and implementing education endeavors that help to improve job performance, enhance organizational effectiveness, and, ultimately, improve patient/family outcomes.

Evidence-based practice (EBP) in staff development focuses on using best practice evidence and identified benchmarks to close the gap between actual staff development practice and identified best practices. We acknowledge the importance of keeping our knowledge of staff development current by reviewing the results of staff development research and implementing, as appropriate, the recommendations identified in such research. We further acknowledge the importance of participating in staff development research and sharing the results of our research with colleagues to enhance the effectiveness of staff development practice.

We respect the dignity, individuality, and cultural beliefs of all learners. Education is planned and delivered within the framework of the principles of adult learning. In order to provide valid and reliable education activities that meet the needs of our learners, we use various teaching/learning methods including, but not limited to, classroom learning, computer-based learning, self-learning initiatives, and other forms of distance education. Teaching/learning methods are continually evaluated for their effectiveness according to the tenants of EBP in staff development. Such evaluation contributes to our body of knowledge and adds to the pool of evidence-based data used to develop staff development products and services.

The staff development department of Manning and Wilson Health System adheres to the following values and principles:

- Learning is a lifelong process.

- Adults are self-directed learners.

- Teaching/learning is a dynamic, interactive process between the learner and the staff development specialist conducted in an environment of mutual respect and regard.

- Adult learners bring a wealth of life experiences to any teaching/learning situation. These experiences facilitate the teaching/learning experience.

- Staff development practice is based on best practice evidence.

- Staff development specialists have a responsibility to contribute to the unique body of knowledge that comprises the specialty of staff development.

Figure 2.3

Sample values statement (cont.)

The staff development specialist is responsible for:

- Establishing a learning environment that adheres to the philosophy of EBP in staff development as well as the principles of adult learning

- Identifying the educational needs of the organization

- Planning education programs based on identified needs of the learners for the purpose of enhancing organizational effectiveness

- Creating education programs that meet the needs of the learners

- Evaluating the effectiveness of education programs as measured by their effect on organizational effectiveness

- Using evaluation data to improve educational activities

- Analyzing evaluation data to contribute to the body of knowledge that is unique to the practice of staff development

Learners are responsible for:

- Identifying their education needs

- Achieving their education goals

- Attending relevant/necessary education programs

- Maintaining competence

- Contributing to the success of education programs

- Evaluating the effectiveness of education programs

- Assuming responsibility for their lifelong learning

Organizational leadership is responsible for:

- Supporting an environment that facilitates lifelong learning

- Collaborating with the staff development department to achieve the organization's education goals

- Facilitating learners' ability to participate in education activities

- Attending relevant or necessary education programs

- Participating in the evaluation of education's impact on organizational effectiveness

- Supporting a learning environment that is based on best practice evidence

Departmental Structure and Description

Departmental structures and descriptions vary widely among organizations. Here are items that should be included in your departmental structure and description.

Structure

- An organizational chart showing the hierarchy and reporting structure of the staff development department. This should include identifying to whom the manager of the staff development department reports.

- Identification of the various roles of the department, a brief description of their duties, and the educational requirements of each. This should not be highly detailed nor should it identify by name who occupies each position. For example, you might identify the role of the NPD specialist by stating: "The department has four NPD specialists who are responsible for the planning, implementation, and evaluation of staff development products and services. Each NPD specialist supervises specific unit-based educators and serves on or chairs specific hospital and nursing councils. The NPD specialist holds a minimum of a master's degree in nursing or a related field." A similar, brief description should be given for each of the department's roles.

Description

- Provide a one- or two-sentence overview of the purpose of your department. For example, you might say that the staff development department "is responsible for the orientation, in-service, and CE of the nursing department. Staff development products and services are evaluated to identify associations between education, patient outcomes, and job performance."

- Identify your customers. For example, do you provide products and services exclusively to the nursing department or are you involved with other departments as well?

- Identify what committees and/or councils are chaired by members of the staff development department. Also note what committees have staff development personnel as members.

- Identify any partnerships or collaborations. These might include online education companies, professional associations, and/or staff development departments from other hospitals or health systems.

Products and Services

Products and services vary among staff development departments. This is the section of your plan where you have an opportunity to explain the nature of your services. Do not go into too much detail—readers will ignore the extra work. Keep this section concise, but be sure to identify your essential products and services such as:

- Orientation for the department of nursing

- Mandatory annual training for the entire hospital

- In-service education and on-the-job training for the department of nursing

- Coordination of student clinical experiences with affiliated schools of nursing (identify universities with which you are affiliated)

- Development, implementation, and ongoing evaluation of nursing preceptorships

- Provision of CE for the department of nursing

These are just some examples of products and services. The point is to tell the readers of your business plan exactly what products and services you provide. Do not go into elaborate detail. The reader is not really interested in details. He or she just wants to get an overview of what it is that you do.

Marketing

Why do you need to worry about marketing staff development products and services? First and foremost, marketing is a way to get your customers (managers, nurses, etc.) to participate in teaching/ learning activities. Failure to market your products and services may have an adverse impact on attendance. Marketing is also a way to generate positive public relations about your department.

This section of your business plan is where you describe how you market your products and services. It should give you a chance to think about some innovative ways to perform this marketing. Here are some examples of marketing tools to include in this section of your business plan:

- **Customer identification:** Who are your customers? For example, are your customers primarily members of the nursing department? Or do you provide services to multiple departments or even the entire organization? Do you have customers external to the organization, such as nurses in a tristate area who are members of a target audience for conferences or distance learning endeavors?

- **Competitor identification:** Who are your competitors? Some online education companies offer CE to organizations at bargain prices. This can actually be competitive if your administration feels that it can outsource CE and decrease the size of your department. Seek out opportunities to collaborate with such companies (e.g., write some CE programs for them) rather than face them as competitors. Identify your competitors and how you plan to decrease the effects of such competition.

- **Education calendar:** Most staff development departments have some type of calendar, often electronic, that identifies what type of education offerings are available, what format those offerings are in, and how to register. Identify these elements in your business plan. Be sure to include how staff members access the calendar. You may also want to identify any thoughts you have on revising the calendar to make it more easily accessible and/or stimulate interest in programs. Illustrations, graphics, and other eye-catching tools are helpful.

                    The Survival of Staff Development

- **Conference announcements:** If your department, alone or in collaboration with other organizations, plans and implements CE conferences, be sure to note this in the marketing section of your business plan. Identify how you market the program, including such items as target audience, a copy of any brochures for the conference(s), and anticipated outcomes such as monetary profit.

- **Collaborations and partnerships:** Describe the nature of any collaborations and/or partnerships. Explain why these are advantageous to your department and how they are marketed to your customers.

- **Marketing outcomes:** Identify what you believe will be the outcomes of your marketing efforts. For example, do you anticipate a monetary profit? Enhanced patient outcomes? Improved job performance? How will you gather evidence to back up your anticipated outcomes?

Action Plan

The action plan tells the reader what you are going to do and when you are going to do it. It assigns responsibility for actions and identifies desired outcomes. Figure 2.4 shows some sample items that might appear in the action plan section of a staff development business plan.

Figure 2.4

Sample action plan

Goal: Become a tristate leader in the provision of continuing education that concentrates on pediatric healthcare services.

Objective(s)	Actions	Responsibility	Target date
• Facilitate achievement of pediatric certification by 90% of RNs working in pediatrics	• Design certification review course	• D. Jones, RN	• December 3, 2010
	• Offer certification review course quarterly	• D. Jones, RN	• February 4, 2011
		• S. Ames, RN	• April 3, 2011
		• K. Eden, RN	• July 10, 2011
		• R. Gordan, RN	• October 14, 2011
• Offer two-day conference on innovations in pediatric surgery	• Conduct needs assessment	• A. Adams, RN	• January 31, 2011
	• Identify target audience and potential participants	• T. Bates, RN	
	• Identify content	• S. Norman, RN	• February 28, 2011
		• P. Sanders, RN	
	• Identify faculty	• M. Mason, RN	• March 30, 2011
		• C. Ames, RN	
	• Design marketing brochure	• M. Simmons, RN	• April 10, 2011
	• Apply for contact hours	• A. Adams, RN	
	• Arrange for conference facilities	• T. Bates, RN	
	• Design evaluation tools, including follow-up process to identify results of education in participants' work settings	• S. Norman, RN	• April 10, 2011
		• P. Sanders, RN	
	• Implement conference	• D. Jones, RN	• September 30, 2011
		• S. Ames, RN	
		• K. Eden, RN	
		• R. Gordan, RN	

The Survival of Staff Development

Budget

The budgetary process involves predicting the cost of salaries, day-to-day operations, and the purchase of major pieces of equipment such as simulation manikins. All organizations have a template that guides the way budgets are prepared. But it's important to include, within that template, justification for expenditures. Here are some ideas for preparing your staff development budget:

- Have you taken into consideration salary increases based not only on merit but on achievement of certification, graduate degrees, or other accomplishments that are linked to monetary rewards?

- When requesting major equipment purchases, have you identified the anticipated impact on your department? For example, if you want to invest in simulation equipment, have you explained how it will enhance learning and job performance? You need to have evidence to back up your requests. In the case of simulation equipment, the literature identifies the positive effects of using such equipment.

- How are you using evidence to justify expenditures? Can you provide evidence that a continued expense, such as computer-based learning, has a positive impact? In other words, have you gathered appropriate data to document knowledge acquisition, on-the-job behaviors, and results (see Chapter 3)?

> **STAFF DEVELOPMENT ALERT!** When preparing your budget, pay attention to any restrictions regarding salaries and projects that correlate with organizational priorities. If limits are placed on you regarding employee salaries and education projects that reflect organizational needs, it may mean that the staff development department is under scrutiny for possible cuts.

Executive Summary

The executive summary, although written last, is usually the first component of a business plan. It is a one- or two-page overview of your complete plan. Use the first paragraph or two of each section of your plan to compile the executive summary.

Often, administrators or busy managers will read only the executive summary of subordinates' business plans. That is why it is so critical that you use the best, most informative, and concise pieces of information from each component of your plan to include in the executive summary. The details of the business plan will guide all members of your department in all of their job-related activities. The person to whom staff development reports will most likely read the entire plan. However, others may only read the executive summary, so be sure it conveys the essence of staff development!

Figure 2.5 offers a review of each component of your business plan. It contains questions to help you be sure that you have included all essential information.

Figure 2.5

Business plan component review

Component	Questions to address
Mission	• Does the staff development's mission coincide with the organization's mission? • Does the mission statement communicate the purpose and direction of the staff development department to those within and outside of the department? • Does the mission statement explain why the staff development department exists?

Vision	• Does the staff development's vision coincide with the organization's vision?
	
	• Is the staff development vision:
	
	  – Clear?
	
	  – Concise?
	
	  – Driven by values?
	
	  – Future-oriented?
	
	  – Inspiring?
	
	  – Realistic?

Values	• Do the staff development values reflect the organizational values? • Does the organizational values statement contain references to the importance of continuing education and lifelong learning? • Have you included references to evidence-based practice in staff development in your values statement? • Have you included references to adult learning principles in your values statement? • Have you identified learner, staff development, and organizational responsibilities as they pertain to education in your values statement?

Figure 2.5

Business plan component review (cont.)

Component	Questions to address

Departmental structure and description	• Have you included an organizational chart of the department?
	
	• Have you explained the various roles in the department?
	
	• Have you identified:
	
	   — Your overall purpose?
	
	   — Your customers?
	
	   — Committee memberships?
	
	   — Partnerships and collaborations?

Products and services	• Have you concisely identified your products and services? • Do these products and services coincide with organizational goals?
Marketing	• Have you identified your customers? • Have you identified your competitors? • How do you compile and distribute the staff development department's education calendar? • How do you describe collaborative marketing efforts? • What are your anticipated marketing outcomes?
Action plan	• Have you identified goals based on organizational goals? • Does each component of the action plan have measurable objectives, specific actions, identified responsibility, and target achievement dates?
Budget	• Have you added monetary increases based on educational achievements? • How have you justified major equipment purchases? • What evidence have you provided to justify expenditures? • Have you been placed on unexpected restrictions when it comes to your budget?
Executive summary	• Have you compiled the critical information from each component of your plan as part of the executive summary?

References

Avillion, A.E. (2008). *A Practical Guide to Staff Development: Evidence-Based Tools and Techniques for Effective Education* (2nd ed.). Marblehead, MA: HCPro.

Golway, M.M. (2009). Purpose, philosophy, and objectives. In S.L. Bruce (Ed.), *Core curriculum for staff development* (3rd ed., pp. 21–32). Pensacola, FL: National Nursing Staff Development Organization.

Hiam, A. (2010). *Business Innovations for Dummies*. Hoboken, NJ: Wiley Publishing.

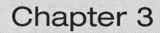

Chapter 3

Linking Evidence-Based Practice in Staff Development to the Five Levels of Evaluation

Linking Evidence-Based Practice in Staff Development to the Five Levels of Evaluation

LEARNING OBJECTIVES

After reading this chapter, you will be able to:

- Explain the concept of evidence-based practice (EBP) in staff development

- Correlate EBP in staff development to departmental and job survival

- Perform all levels of program evaluation from the perspective of EBP in staff development

Introduction

Evidence-based practice (EBP) in staff development is the ongoing analysis of education to identify best practices and benchmarks. The implementation of best practices and benchmarks should help to close the gap between actual staff development practice and identified best practices (Avillion, 2007).

The use of evidence to identify best practices and benchmarks relies on gathering data from a variety of sources and objectively analyzing that data to garner such evidence. The ultimate goal of the staff development department is to use evidence to develop educational products and services that enhance job performance and improve patient outcomes.

But what kinds of evidence do we need to demonstrate an association between education and improved patient outcomes and job performance? All too often, we gather data only about participants' reactions, knowledge gain, and learner behaviors in the work setting. That is not to say that these kinds of data are unimportant—they are very important.

However, they are not important enough to show the true value of the staff development department without also performing results-oriented evaluation.

Evidence-Based Practice in Staff Development and Job Survival

EBP is implemented to close the gap between actual staff development practice and identified best practices. The rationale behind EBP is to show a positive association between education and desired patient outcomes and job performance. But how does EBP affect job survival for the individual staff development practitioner?

In the clinical setting, nurses' job performance evaluations are based, in large part, on patient outcomes. In the staff development setting, practitioners' job performance evaluations should be based, in large part, on the impact of the educational activities they plan and implement.

No one is guaranteed a job or continued employment. However, if you can demonstrate a link between educational products and services that you develop and a positive impact on the organization, you stand a better chance of surviving when position and budget cuts threaten the staff development department. In other words, you are demonstrating your value in measurable ways.

The most obvious way to demonstrate these kinds of links is with specific education programs. Suppose you have made specific revisions to your facility's nursing orientation. By comparing evidence such as turnover, length of retention following orientation, and preceptor evaluations of orientees before and after these revisions, you may be able to demonstrate a link between your revisions and positive change in these areas: a decrease in turnover, an increase in retention, and/or more favorable preceptor evaluations of employees.

Another example is related to interpersonal communication skills, which can be a challenge in most organizations. An increase in patient complaints and/or reports of peer bullying trigger the need for education. Comparing data pertaining to patient complaints and/or reports of peer bullying before and after you implement an interpersonal communication skills program can help to show an association between your initiatives and positive outcomes.

Do not limit your evidence strictly to education programs, though. Nursing professional development (NPD) specialists are valuable members of hospital councils and committees, and are often called on to assume the role of chairpersons. Look at how the goals and objectives of councils and committees are achieved, and be able to address the following questions:

- What part did you play in these achievements? Can you trace specific actions you took that were instrumental to the success of these groups? What was the impact on the organization following achievement of council and committee goals and objectives?

- Have you published articles that highlighted your achievements or contributions to staff development? What kind of positive publicity did your department and organization receive as a result of your publishing efforts?

- Have you presented a paper or poster at a local or national convention or conference? Did you make sure that you, your department, and your organization received positive publicity from your presentation(s)?

- Does your supervisor and administration know that you published and/or presented and that the organization received favorable publicity as a result of your efforts? Include these kinds of achievements in your monthly reports or whatever means you have of communicating your accomplishments.

Take a long, hard look at what you do and how you can objectively demonstrate that your actions have a positive impact on both your department and your organization. Make sure that your achievements are known to supervisors and administration. Although there is no foolproof way to guarantee job security, keeping track of how you as an individual improve departmental and organizational effectiveness is an important strategy when looking for ways to make your position a strong one that is necessary in your organization.

Evidence-Based Practice in Staff Development and Departmental Survival

Your department's survival depends on its demonstrated positive impact on the organization. This impact can only be demonstrated if every member of the department participates in EBP and is aware of the consequences of failing to implement it.

The need for all members of the department to "buy in" to the concept of EBP in staff development is essential. As previously mentioned, EBP must be incorporated into your mission, vision, and values statements. All members of the department must receive education and training in the concept of EBP in staff development, and, more importantly, understand how its implementation helps improve the odds of staff development survival.

EBP allows you and your staff development colleagues to objectively demonstrate that what you do (and how you do it) really does make a difference to patient outcomes and job performance. Share the impact of education at every opportunity. Although nothing can guarantee absolute departmental protection from position and budget cuts, a department that has a measurable positive impact is less likely to be scrutinized.

As with individual staff development specialist job performance, the most obvious way to demonstrate impact is through education offerings. The link between education, patient outcomes, and job performance is the most effective way to enhance departmental survival. However, do not neglect other aspects of staff development responsibilities.

As previously mentioned, individual members of the staff development department are members of or chair a variety of organizational hospitals and committees. Make sure everyone, both members and chairpersons, knows that they should be documenting how their performance contributes to the department and organization. The ultimate goal is to show that they (and the staff development department they represent) are crucial to achievement of council and committee objectives, and that such achievement is critical to the organization.

Positive publicity for the staff development department is essential to its survival. Make sure that if the members of the department are publishing and presenting, these accomplishments are noted in the organization's publications, such as newsletters, and on the organization's website.

Ultimately, survival depends on how well you show that the staff development department is essential to organizational functioning. You can produce evidence to this effect by gathering and analyzing data carefully and systematically. A process must be in place for these actions. One way (and perhaps the most practical way) to produce evidence is to develop a system based on the five levels of evaluation commonly used by staff development personnel.

The Levels of Evaluation and Evidence-Based Practice in Staff Development

Most NPD specialists are familiar with the evaluation model based on Kirkpatrick's (1994) work on program evaluation. The model consists of five levels of evaluation:

- Reaction

- Knowledge acquisition or learning

- Behavior

- Results

- Return on investment (ROI)

It is important that initial levels such as reaction be used as a foundation for succeeding levels. Data should never be gathered from one level and used in isolation from the others. Here are some suggestions for gathering and analyzing data from each level and incorporating analysis into EBP in staff development.

Reaction

Reactive data are used to assess learner satisfaction or "reaction" to a teaching/learning activity (Kirkpatrick, 1994). Sometimes referred to as a "happiness" index, these data indicate satisfaction (or dissatisfaction) with the teaching method, the learning environment, how well the learners felt they were able to achieve learning objectives, and how effective they thought the teacher was.

Figures 3.1 and 3.2 are sample templates for gathering reactive data in the classroom setting and from distance learning activities.

> **STAFF DEVELOPMENT ALERT!** Learners' reactions are important. However, these data cannot be used in isolation to gather evidence. Data should be used as a basis for succeeding levels of evaluation.

How can you use reactive data to promote staff development activities? Here are some examples:

Caroline is responsible for the implementation of education to help nurses and other emergency department personnel deal with verbally and physically violent patients and families. The classroom component is always held in the same location due to space and equipment needs. This classroom is in an older part of the hospital with inadequate heat in the winter and not enough air conditioning in the summer. Participants complain that they hate attending class because the environment is so uncomfortable. Caroline has been advocating for additional classroom space that is more conducive to learning. How can she use these initial reaction data to achieve her goal?

Although learner comfort is important, their discomfort is not enough to convince administration that additional classroom space is necessary. Caroline can use these data as a starting point, however. With the data, she can answer these questions to determine how to proceed:

- Has the discomfort of the learning environment led to a decrease in attendance?

- Has the discomfort of the learning environment interfered with the ability of the participants to learn, as evidenced by posttest scores or skill demonstrations?

- Has the discomfort of the learning environment led to a decrease in the ability of staff members to effectively deal with aggressive patients and families?

Figure 3.1

Classroom evaluation form

Date: _____

Time: _____

Name (optional): _____

Department and unit: _____

Title: _____ (e.g., RN)

Program title: _____

Instructor(s): _____

Objectives: 1. _____

           2. _____

           3. _____

Please answer the following questions by checking the response that best describes your feelings. (Note: N/A stands for non-applicable.)

1. How well did the program content meet the stated objectives?

        __Excellent __Very good __Good __Fair __Poor __N/A

2. Based on the program content, how well were you able to achieve the objectives?

        a. Objective #1 _____

        __Excellent __Very good __Good __Fair __Poor __N/A

        b. Objective #2 _____

        __Excellent __Very good __Good __Fair __Poor __N/A

        c. Objective #3 _____

        __Excellent __Very good __Good __Fair __Poor __N/A

3. Did this program offer information that will help you to do your job?

        __Yes __No

        Please explain: _____

        _____

        _____

4. Was the instructor(s) an effective teacher?

        __Excellent __Very good __Good __Fair __Poor __N/A

Figure 3.1

Classroom evaluation form (cont.)

5. Was the instructor(s) knowledgeable and well prepared to teach this program?

__Excellent __Very good __Good __Fair __Poor __N/A

6. Was there enough time for discussion and to ask questions?

__Excellent __Very good __Good __Fair __Poor __N/A

7. Did the instructor show respect for the participants?

__Excellent __Very good __Good __Fair __Poor __N/A

8. Were your questions answered to your satisfaction?

__Yes __No

Please explain. _____

_____

_____

9. Were the handouts useful?

__Excellent __Very good __Good __Fair __Poor __N/A

10. Were you able to read the handouts without difficulty?

__Excellent __Very good __Good __Fair __Poor __N/A

11. Were the audiovisuals (A/V) useful?

__Excellent __Very good __Good __Fair __Poor __N/A

12. Was the temperature of the classroom comfortable?

__Excellent __Very good __Good __Fair __Poor __N/A

13. Were the seating arrangements comfortable?

__Excellent __Very good __Good __Fair __Poor __N/A

14. Were you able to see and hear the instructor without difficulty?

__Excellent __Very good __Good __Fair __Poor __N/A

Figure 3.1

Classroom evaluation form (cont.)

15. Were you able to see and hear the A/Vs used without difficulty?

__Excellent __Very good __Good __Fair __Poor __N/A

16. Additional comments:

_____

_____

_____

_____

17. For future program planning, please identify three specific education topics that would help you improve your ability to do your job.

1. _____

2. _____

3. _____

18. What would be the most efficient, convenient way for you to attend programs focusing on the topics you identified above? If you choose more than one format, please rank them in order of preference with 1 being the most preferred, 2 the second most preferred, etc.

Classroom _____   Audio conference _____

Self-learning modules _____   Teleconferencing _____

DVD _____   Computer-based learning _____

Closed-circuit television _____   Audiotape _____

Web seminar _____

Other (please identify): _____

_____

_____

Source: This tool was adapted from The Practical Guide to Staff Development, *Second Edition (2008), by Adrianne E. Avillion, DEd, RN.*

Figure 3.2	

Distance learning evaluation form

Date: _____

Time: _____

Name (optional): _____

Department and unit: _____

Title: _____ (e.g., RN)

Program title: _____

Teaching method (Please check all that apply):

     ___ Computer-based learning   ___ Web seminar   ___ DVD

     ___ Self-learning packet   ___ Audiotape   ___ Teleconference

     ___ Closed-circuit television   ___ Audio conference

     Other (please identify): _____

                     _____

                     _____

Objectives: 1. _____

          2. _____

          3. _____

Please answer the following questions. (Note: N/A stands for non-applicable.)

1. How well did the program content meet the stated objectives?

     __Excellent __Very good __Good __Fair __Poor __N/A

2. Based on the program content, how well were you able to achieve the objectives?

     a. Objective #1 _____

     __Excellent __Very good __Good __Fair __Poor __N/A

     b. Objective #2 _____

     __Excellent __Very good __Good __Fair __Poor __N/A

     c. Objective #3 _____

     __Excellent __Very good __Good __Fair __Poor __N/A

Figure 3.2

Distance learning evaluation form (cont.)

3. Did this program offer information that will help you to do your job?

__Yes   __No

Please explain: _____

_____

_____

_____

4. Was the teaching method effective?

__Excellent __Very good __Good __Fair __Poor __N/A

5. How well were you able to use the equipment for this distance learning experience?

__Excellent __Very good __Good __Fair __Poor __N/A

6. How well did the program explain how to receive help or to ask questions if necessary?

__Excellent __Very good __Good __Fair __Poor __N/A

7. Were the handouts useful?

__Excellent __Very good __Good __Fair __Poor __N/A

8. Were you able to read the handouts without difficulty?

__Excellent __Very good __Good __Fair __Poor __N/A

9. Was the equipment needed to participate in this program in good working order?

__Yes   __No

Please explain. _____

_____

_____

10. Was the location of this distance learning experience quiet and comfortable?

__Excellent __Very good __Good __Fair __Poor __N/A

Figure 3.2

Distance learning evaluation form (cont.)

11. If you had questions about the program or its content, did you receive satisfactory answers?

__Yes __No

Please explain. _____

_____

_____

12. Did the quality of the graphics, videos, or audiotapes help you to learn?

__Excellent __Very good __Good __Fair __Poor __N/A

13. Additional comments:

_____

_____

_____

_____

14. For future program planning, please identify three specific education topics that would help you to improve your ability to do your job.

1. _____

2. _____

3. _____

15. What would be the most efficient, convenient way for you to participate in programs focusing on the topics you identified above? If you choose more than one format, please rank them in order of preference with 1 being the most preferred, 2 the second most preferred, etc.

Classroom _____ Audio conference _____

Self-learning modules _____ Teleconferencing _____

DVD _____ Computer-based learning _____

Closed-circuit television _____ Audiotape _____

Other (please identify): _____

_____

Source: This tool was adapted from The Practical Guide to Staff Development, *Second Edition (2008), by Adrianne E. Avillion, DEd, RN.*

Of course, environment alone cannot be blamed for negative outcomes, but it can certainly contribute to them. Caroline can use reactive data to help determine what impact, if any, the environment has had on desired results.

Here is another example:

> *Jason is responsible for the design and implementation of the nurse preceptor education and training program. This program is quite extensive and has been associated with a decrease in turnover. Two experienced preceptors help Jason teach the course. One preceptor, Monica, has a lively and engaging teaching style and incorporates personal anecdotes and jokes into her presentation delivery. The other preceptor, Opal, has a more formal teaching style and is rather reserved in manner. Both are highly respected by their colleagues as experienced clinicians. Reactive data show that participants prefer Monica to Opal as an instructor. They make multiple positive comments about Monica's lively personality, which they say makes learning fun. Based on these reactive data, a colleague new to staff development asks Jason why he doesn't exclude Opal from participating in the preceptor training. How do you think Jason should reply?*

Less experienced staff development specialists often have a "knee-jerk" response to reactive data. Jason knows that he must carefully evaluate reactive data in conjunction with other types of evaluation findings. Questions he should ask himself include:

- Do learning outcomes differ depending on whether Monica or Opal is teaching the preceptor course?

- Is there a difference in knowledge acquisition?

- Is there a difference in behavior?

- Is there a difference in results?

- Would Monica have time to be the only nurse preceptor involved in teaching the course?

- Is it possible to work with Opal to enhance her presentation style?

Jason knows that more analysis is needed. As an experienced staff development specialist, he knows that reactive data must be evaluated in conjunction with outcomes.

Knowledge acquisition or learning

Learning evaluation measures the extent to which participants gain knowledge. Learning objectives provide the basis for evaluating learning. For example, if your objectives focus on the achievement of intellectual, didactic knowledge, then a written test may be an effective way to measure learning. If the objective is to achieve competence in a specific psychomotor skill, then demonstration of that skill is necessary (Avillion, 2008).

At first glance, it appears that learning data are the easiest to measure. For example, a pretest measures knowledge before education, and a posttest measures knowledge after education is completed. A skill demonstration clarifies whether knowledge has been acquired in the form of a psychomotor skill.

But if EBP is truly a part of your everyday professional life, you need to look at some of the pitfalls of assessing learning. Let's start with probably the most common format: written testing. Consider the following issues as you implement testing as a form of evaluating knowledge acquisition:

- How valid and reliable are your pre- and posttests? Have you assessed the results to determine whether they are actually useful?

- How do learners react to pretests? Some may view them as embarrassing because the purpose of a pretest is to determine what is *not* known. If you are using both pre- and posttests, you need to make it clear to learners that the purpose is to demonstrate knowledge gain, not advertise knowledge gaps.

- Is fear a factor? Passing a specific test may be a requirement of employment. This is the case for critical care nurses who must be Advanced Cardiac Life Support certified or patient care providers who must be certified in CPR. In these cases, fear may interfere with an employee's ability to take a written exam.

- How do you protect the confidentiality of the answers to a written exam? Are employees willing to share information about an exam with friends? If written exams are part of computer-based learning, how have you protected unauthorized access to tests and their answers?

The Survival of Staff Development

These are just some of the issues involved with testing. This is not to say that written testing should be eliminated. It just means that when you gather data to measure learning, you need to be aware of pitfalls as well as strengths.

There may be even more pitfalls when skill demonstration is part of the assessment of knowledge acquisition. Under normal circumstances, more than one person evaluates the performance of a psychomotor skill. How do you ensure that all evaluators are assessing performance in the same way?

Figure 3.3 suggests a template for assessing competency in a psychomotor skill. Note that this template not only includes space for objectives but for the exact steps or actions that the learner must demonstrate to achieve competency. Both the learner and the observer must sign the form indicating that competency was achieved. If competency was not achieved, there is space for a remediation plan as well as space to note the date by which the plan must be implemented. Again, both observer and learner must sign that competency was not achieved. Their signatures are also required to indicate agreement with the plan for remediation.

> **STAFF DEVELOPMENT ALERT!** Signatures have a way of increasing the seriousness of achieving competency. When both parties are required to sign a document, they are more likely to do their best as a learner or an evaluator.

Behavior

Behavioral evaluation is the process of assessing learners' behavior and the actual use of new knowledge/skills during on-the-job performance (Avillion, 2008). By this point in the evidence gathering process, you have gathered data pertaining to learners' reactions and to their knowledge acquisition. Now it is time to determine whether they are correctly applying newly learned behaviors in the work setting.

Gathering evidence of behavioral changes often consists of audits or direct observation. For example, nursing documentation may be reviewed to assess appropriate charting of new procedures. Direct observation of psychomotor skills or communication interventions are ways to gather evidence pertaining to behavior.

The biggest challenge to gathering accurate behavioral evidence is ensuring consistency of evaluation. In almost all instances, more than one person is assessing behavior. How do you know everyone is performing behavioral evaluation in the same way? To ensure consistent behavioral evaluation, templates such as Figures 3.3 and 3.4 should be used by evaluators.

Figure 3.3 can be adapted to accommodate reviewers who are auditing, charting, or observing specific skills. Use of such a template not only helps to ensure consistency of evaluation but avoids accusations of favoritism or inconsistency of approach.

Figure 3.4 offers another template option. It includes space for a variety of behaviors.

STAFF DEVELOPMENT ALERT! Note that in Figure 3.4, space is allotted for specific behaviors as well as objectives. There are also places for the signatures of the person performing the evaluation and the person who is being evaluated.

Behavioral evaluation should be performed by someone who is trained to perform the evaluation process. Whenever possible, avoid having friends evaluate friends and having peers from the same unit evaluate each other. The evaluator should be as objective as possible.

Figure 3.3

Competency assessment

Demonstration of competency achievement

Date: _____   Competency: _____

Objectives: _____

_____

Competency demonstration:

Step 1: _____

Step 2: _____

Step 3: _____

Step 4: _____

Observer comments:

_____

_____

_____

Learner comments:

_____

Competency was achieved: _____   _____

Observer's signature and date   Learner's signature and date

Competency was not achieved: _____   _____

Observer's signature and date   Learner's signature and date

The following steps will be taken by the learner to achieve competency:

_____

_____

These steps will be taken by the following date: _____

Observer's signature

_____

Learner's signature

Source: This tool was adapted from The Practical Guide to Staff Development, *Second Edition (2008), by Adrianne E. Avillion, DEd, RN.*

| Figure 3.4 | Behavioral assessment |

Date: _____

Time: _____

Name and title of person being evaluated: _____

Name and title of person conducting evaluation: _____

Behavior being evaluated:

           _____ Medical record review   _____ Equipment use

           _____ Psychomotor skill   _____ Communication

           _____ Other

Objectives: _____

_____

_____

Specific behaviors that must be noted: _____

_____

_____

Results of evaluation: _____

_____

_____

Were all necessary behaviors present and accurate? _____Yes _____No

If no, explain any omissions or inaccuracies: _____

_____

_____

Were objectives achieved? _____Yes _____No

If no, explain which objectives were not met and why they were not met:

_____

_____

_____

Figure 3.4	Behavioral assessment (cont.)

Evaluator's comments: _____

_____

_____

Remedial action plan if necessary: _____

_____

_____

_____	_____
Evaluator's signature and date	Learner's signature and date

Results

Results indicate outcomes that occurred because of education (Kirkpatrick, 1994). Results are what can give a staff development department the strength and vitality to avoid budget cuts and down-sizing. EBP in staff development relies on obtaining and analyzing data to determine the evidence that exists to link education to job performance and patient outcomes.

When determining this link, be sure to look at the levels of evaluation that preceded results. Suppose you change the format of an education program from classroom style to distance learning format to save time and money, and to avoid having staff members leave their respective units. Learners object, stating that they miss having the opportunity to interact with their peers and enjoy in-person learning. However, on analysis, you find that learning, behavior, and results are the same with distance learning as they were via the classroom format. You need to share these results with learners (and whoever else is affected by the change). It may not make them like the distance learning format, but it will help them to understand your decision.

A good example of linking education to positive results is the implementation of a preceptor training program. Consider this scenario:

> *Jennifer is a newly hired NPD specialist who works in a 500-bed medical center. Prior to her arrival, preceptor training consisted of an overview of adult learning principles and the competencies newly hired nurses must achieve to successfully complete their orientation. All RNs were expected to take turns functioning as preceptors. Turnover within the first year of hire for newly licensed nurses was nearly 70%. During exit interviews, the majority of nurses cited poor preceptorship as a major reason for their resignations. Jennifer is assigned to fix the preceptor program. Keeping in mind that EBP in staff development is the foundation of her practice, how should Jennifer proceed?*

Jennifer needs to gather data pertaining to reaction, learning, behavior, and results before designing a preceptor program. What kinds of evidence should she obtain? The following is a list of specific evidence she should collect from each evaluation level before proceeding:

- **Reactive data:** Review the data newly hired nurses completed regarding orientation, especially their interactions with preceptors. Is there a pattern to positive reactions as well as negative reactions? Are there particular preceptors who receive more negative comments compared to others? What do the data from exit interviews indicate about preceptors? Ask all preceptors to complete (if they have not already done so) an evaluation of their training as preceptors.

> **STAFF DEVELOPMENT ALERT!** Not everyone is cut out to be a preceptor! Preceptors should want to assume this role. It should be part of an organization's career advancement program, along with appropriate education and training and monetary rewards.

- **Learning:** What do data indicate regarding learning? Is there a pattern to learning, especially as it relates to competencies? What is the content of the current preceptor training? What is lacking?

- **Behavior:** Is there a pattern to orientees' achievement of (or failure to achieve) required competencies during orientation? Is there a link between failures to achieve competency and preceptors assigned to the orientees who fail?

- **Results:** What impact is the preceptor program having on the organization? What is the turn-over rate? Is it linked to specific preceptors? What is the cost of the turnover in terms of orienting nurses who leave within the first year and of having to replace them?

Only after Jennifer has the answers to these questions can she begin to revise preceptor education and training. She will probably make recommendations concerning how preceptors are selected, trained, and rewarded. She will also most likely change the content and length of preceptor education and training. Additionally, she should identify the desired results of these revisions, such as decreasing turnover to 20% within a reasonable period of time.

After making revisions to the content of preceptor training and, in conjunction with the nurse managers and nursing administration, making changes to preceptor selection, Jennifer will implement her revised education and training for preceptors. She will need to gather the same kinds of data identified previously and compare results.

Figure 3.5 is a sample template to use when preparing to gather evidence related to results. Note that there is space for summaries of the levels preceding results. You cannot analyze results in isolation from other data any more than you can rely solely on reaction or learning data. Remember that your ultimate goal is to be able to analyze results for the purpose of providing evidence that links education to improvements in patient outcomes, job performance, and/or organizational effectiveness.

Figure 3.5

Results data gathering

Level of evaluation	Summary of data	Conclusions/actions
Reaction		
Learning		
Behavior		
Results		

Return on investment

Return on investment (ROI) is a measure, in terms of dollars and cents, of the financial impact of education efforts. Monetary evidence is always compelling, especially in an era of ongoing economic crises. Measurement of ROI should be reserved for major programs that cost a significant amount of money, such as orientation or, if your organization plans such events, conferences that attract a significant audience from a broad geographic location.

A simple formula that you can use to calculate ROI as a percentage is:

$$\text{ROI (\%)} = \frac{\text{Net program benefits}}{\text{Program costs}} \times 100$$

ROI can also be calculated as a simple dollar amount. For example, determine the ROI of orientation including (Avillion, 2008):

- Turnover

- The costs of overtime by current employees to cover extra shifts until new employees have completed orientation

- The costs in terms of salary for staff development personnel and preceptors to provide orientation and on-the-job supervision

- The costs in terms of salary for staff development personnel to plan, implement, and evaluate orientation

- The costs of supplies, equipment, etc., used for orientation

If you are revising orientation and/or preceptor programs, compare these costs before and after implementing any revisions.

As noted, it is not realistic to expect that you will calculate ROI on every education program you implement. However, it is important that you identify those programs for which ROI is essential. Here are some tips for selecting education products and services for which you should calculate ROI:

- Any program that is a collaborative education effort. Such efforts include education conferences conducted with colleagues from other organizations and/or colleges and universities. These kinds of programs generate significant expenses, including speaker fees, marketing materials, staff time to deal with registrations, meals, etc. Income should at least equal expenses. In some cases, especially if you are trying to establish a reputation as a host of major conferences, it may be necessary to generate significant profit. One of the first steps when planning these types of collaborative efforts is to determine whether making a profit is a priority objective, and what the profit will be used for.

- Programs which are crucial to organizational survival. Orientation is a good example. The costs of orienting new employees are considerable, as is the cost of turnover. ROI should be considered a necessity for your orientation program.

- Programs relating to accreditation status. For example, you should calculate the costs of programs that involve preparing staff for visits by accrediting agencies such as The Joint Commission. Many organizations are pursuing various specialty certifications such as trauma centers, stroke centers, and/or ANCC Magnet Recognition® (MRP) status. You need to know the monetary cost of education related to accreditation preparation because in these cases, success is not measured by the "income" from accreditation—it is measured by successful achievement of accreditation. You need to be able to show that expenses related to education and training are well worth the money.

- Any endeavor that involves consultative services. Have you hired consultants regarding specific education needs, such as nursing competency programs or MRP survey preparedness? You need to be able to justify these kinds of expenses. Perhaps the ROI cannot be measured in monetary terms, but it can be measured in other ways such as achieving the desired goals of hiring a consultant.

- Any program that requires use of grant money. Many organizations pursue grants for specific projects, especially those related on clinical research. Grant applications require detailed descriptions of how any funds will be used. Your organization will want to know how and why grant money was spent and what the ROI is.

In summary, EBP depends on gathering data from the first four levels of evaluation on a consistent basis. Demonstrating that the results of staff development products and services have a positive monetary impact on the organization enhances the quality of your department and decreases the danger of yourself or your department experiencing cuts in budget and positions.

References

Avillion, A.E. (2007). *Evidence-Based Staff Development: Strategies to Create, Measure, and Refine Your Program*. Marblehead, MA: HCPro.

Avillion, A.E. (2008). *A Practical Guide to Staff Development: Evidence-Based Tools and Techniques for Effective Education* (2nd ed.). Marblehead, MA: HCPro.

Kirkpatrick, D.L. (1994). *Evaluating Training Programs: The Four Levels*. San Francisco: Berrett-Koehler Publishers.

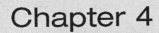

Chapter 4

Linking Evidence-Based Practice in Staff Development to Specific Products and Services

CHAPTER 4

Linking Evidence-Based Practice in Staff Development to Specific Products and Services

Introduction

Evidence-based practice (EBP) in staff development is the foundation of practice. Whether we are planning and implementing a complex continuing education program, an in-service, or just-in-time training, EBP is our base.

EBP can also be applied to our contributions to achievement of accreditation, committee and council participation, and indeed, all of our staff development endeavors. This chapter focuses on the application of EBP to specific staff development products and services.

Orientation

Orientation seems to be in a constant state of flux. For orientees, orientation is never long enough, and for managers, preceptors, and staff members, it is never short enough. We seem to be bombarded by requests to change orientation on an almost daily basis. Responding to these requests is time-consuming and frustrating. The best way to deal with these kinds of issues is to rely on evidence to support change or to justify maintenance.

Evidence is the product of an ongoing, systematic analysis of a specific product—in this case, orientation. If you are considering changing orientation—for example, shifting the format from classroom to distance learning—conduct a pilot study first. Compare results (e.g., competency, learning) of both formats before making a final decision. You need evidence that will support your decision to change or maintain the format of your orientation program.

The first column in Figure 4.1 is for the identification of a specific component of orientation such as documentation, medication administration, mandatory training, etc. Look at each facet of orientation and the teaching/learning methodology (identified in the second column) for each. For example, you might want to analyze documentation, for which your teaching/learning methodology is a combination of classroom instruction and computer-based learning. Next, you would document in the evaluation data summary column a statement or two that summarizes the results of each level of evaluation.

The evidence column allows you to document the evidence you have identified from your evaluation analysis. For instance, reaction data might be summarized as "80% of participants stated that the blended learning format was helpful. Twenty percent stated that they would have preferred an all-classroom-style format." Your evidence would focus on the overall results of this particular orientation component, such as "Documentation audits showed that 90% of new orientees' documentation met stated objectives of appropriate nursing documentation. During a recent Joint Commission survey, the surveyor complimented new orientees' documentation skills and noted this in survey results."

Examine the data from each level of evaluation. Determine whether there are any links between the various levels, and what those links are. For instance, do reaction data indicate a profound dislike of a particular teaching method? Is this supported by a lack of learning, behavior, or results?

> **STAFF DEVELOPMENT ALERT!** Remember, you cannot analyze levels of evaluation in isolation from one another!

After your analysis of evaluation data, what evidence have you identified? Does the evidence support what you are doing, or does it indicate a need for change?

 The Survival of Staff Development

Figure 4.1

Orientation analysis

Orientation component	Teaching/learning methodology	Evaluation data summary	Evidence
		Reaction: Learning: Behavior: Results: Return on investment:	

When evaluating orientation, you must include the following:

- **Turnover**: Is turnover roughly equal on all units, or are particular units experiencing more turnover than others?

- **Preceptors**: Is turnover linked to specific preceptors? What does analysis of your preceptor program tell you about possible links to retention and turnover?

> **STAFF DEVELOPMENT ALERT!** Figure 4.1 can be adapted to analyze your preceptor program. Simply substitute the term "Preceptor program component" for "Orientation component" in the first column.

- **Costs**: What is the cost of orienting a new employee in your organization? Work with human resources to determine the cost by calculating salaries of new employees, preceptors, staff development personnel, etc. Although there is no fixed figure for the costs of orientation, it can be as high as $50,000 per new employee.

Whatever method you choose to analyze orientation, be sure that it is done in a systematic manner and on an ongoing basis (e.g., quarterly). Use a template adapted to the needs of your organization to help you organize findings in a consistent manner.

In-Service Education

In-service education generally refers to simple, short-term programming that meets an immediate need. In-service education is often a swift response to a change in your work environment; for example, it might cover how to quickly learn how to use new equipment (Avillion, 2008).

When multiple learners must achieve competency right away, a template for documentation, such as the example in Figure 4.2, is helpful. This template allows the instructor to easily document the achievement of many learners.

Using templates can help you to document and retrieve data fairly easily. However, what about when problems arise with the demand for in-services? How can you use EBP to justify a change in the number and/or frequency of in-services? An example follows.

Allison is a unit-based educator who is responsible for in-service implementation on three medical units. Over the past 12 months, vendors with new equipment have impressed several prominent physicians, as well as administration. As a result, new equipment seems to arrive several times per month, along with demands by physicians and administration that all nurses become competent in the use of this new equipment. However, the patient population seldom requires these new devices. As a result, nurses are continually being in-serviced on equipment that they rarely, if ever, see again. What kinds of evidence should Allison gather to help put a stop to this problem?

Figure 4.2

In-service template for new equipment

Competency: _____

Objectives: _____

_____

_____

Instructor's name and title: _____

The following persons have achieved competency in the use of

_____ by demonstrating achievement of the stated objectives.

	Date	Time	Learner's signature and title
1.			
2.			
3.			
4.			
5.			
6.			

_____

Instructor's signature and date

All educators know that in order to remain competent in a specific skill, nurses must have the opportunity to implement that skill in the work setting. It is not enough to explain this to the physicians and administration in this example. Allison needs evidence. Some steps she could take include:

- Determining the time it takes her to provide these kinds of in-services and, based on her hourly salary, calculating how much it costs her to provide them.

- Determining the time and cost of in-servicing all nurses. To do this, Allison may need to obtain an average wage for nurses as she will likely not have access to each nurse's salary information.

- Determining how much of the new equipment, if any, was used after in-services were provided.

- Determining the cost of purchasing or renting equipment that was rarely, if ever, used.

Once she has taken the above steps, Allison can present administration with time and money as evidence. This may not completely stop the problem, but it will probably help to decrease the frequency of its occurrence. The point, for Allison and for all of us, is to think in terms of evidence.

Continuing Education

Continuing education is usually referred to as learning activities designed to augment an employee's professional growth and development (Avillion, 2008). The provision of continuing education has changed drastically in the last few years. Once primarily a classroom phenomenon, continuing education is now offered via a myriad of technological entities such as Web seminars, computer-based learning, and teleconferencing. As mentioned in Chapter 3, results are what we are most interested in when it comes to proving our value to the organization.

You should always think in terms of evidence related to results when planning continuing education programs. When identifying learning objectives, think of how achievement of these objectives will impact job performance and/or patient outcomes.

Let's take another look at the template in Figure 4.1 and adapt it to continuing education in Figure 4.3.

Figure 4.3

Continuing education analysis

Continuing education program	How learning objectives will show results	Evaluation data summary	Evidence
		Reaction: Learning: Behavior: Results: Return on investment:	

Note that the second column focuses on how the learning objectives show results. By including this type of terminology in a template, you will be forced to think about results-oriented data when you are writing your learning objectives. For example, if a program on rehabilitation of stroke patients is being evaluated, results might include a decrease in length of stay or improved independence in activities of daily living (ADL) following rehabilitation. The evidence could be documented in the exact length of stay for the stroke population or outcomes calculated on ADL scales.

Accreditation, Committees and Councils, and External Accomplishments as They Relate to Evidence-Based Practice in Staff Development

As noted in previous chapters, we need to think about our work on committees and councils in terms of evidence and how that evidence can help demonstrate our value to the organization. We are members of or chair many of the most critical committees, councils, and task forces of the organization. Here are some suggestions regarding linking evidence to our performance as members or chairpersons of these important entities:

- **Accreditation:** What responsibilities do you have for accreditation efforts? Regardless of the particular accreditation being sought, you need to document what specific contributions you (and members of the staff development department) have made to achieving accreditation. What kinds of education have you implemented to facilitate accreditation achievement? What were the results of that education? Make sure that you report the evidence that links results to education during meetings that focus on accreditation preparation. Never hesitate to share this type of evidence!

- **Committees and councils:** What committees and councils do staff development personnel chair? On what committees and councils do they serve as members? How are you documenting evidence of your contributions? For example, suppose the risk management/quality improvement council identifies specific problems that require education. Common problems include infection rates, falls, and patient complaints. After the implementation of appropriate education, problems resolve or decrease in severity. Make sure that you report these results during meetings, and be sure that these results are recorded in the minutes of the council or committee! This provides a written record of your evidence.

- **Publications and presentations:** Many nursing professional development (NPD) specialists and other members of the staff development department have published articles in professional journals. They have also presented, via papers and/or posters, at conventions and conferences. These kinds of accomplishments serve as excellent publicity for the person involved, her or his department, and the organization. How are you communicating these accomplishments? They should be documented in departmental meeting minutes and as part of the reporting mechanism to the person who oversees the manager of the staff development department. These accomplishments should also be reported at appropriate committee and council meetings. Suppose you have published an article on innovations in preceptor programs. Make sure that you share this during nurse manager meetings/councils. If you present a paper on how education helped to decrease patient complaints, make sure that the risk management/quality improvement committee knows about your presentation and that it is documented in the minutes.

> **STAFF DEVELOPMENT ALERT!** Never miss an opportunity to share evidence of your value to the organization! Do not be shy! The only way to enhance your viability is to share your achievements!

Figure 4.4 is a sample accomplishment template. This should help keep you on track when reporting your achievements. The first column identifies specific tasks such as council membership. The second column is for documentation of the accomplishment(s) related to the identified task. Finally, the third column identifies exactly how these accomplishments were reported.

This kind of template is one way of helping you to communicate your EBP findings to the organization. Let's look at some additional methods and tips for communicating your achievements in the following section.

Figure 4.4

Sample task accomplishment template

Task	Evidence of accomplishments	Reporting mechanism
Member of risk management/quality improvement council	20% reduction in fall rate following safety education and training	1. Reported findings during council meeting 2. Recorded evidence in council meeting minutes 3. Documented in monthly departmental minutes 4. Reported to vice president for clinical services during monthly meeting

Communicating Evidence-Based Practice Findings to Management and Administration

Communicate with confidence in person

The first, and arguably the most important, principle of good communication is to communicate your evidence with confidence. Far too many NPD specialists are afraid that communicating their accomplishments will seem like bragging. Failure to communicate increases your vulnerability to downsizing and budget cuts!

Confidence, when communicating in person, should incorporate the following components:

- **Be prepared.** Use whatever template works best for you to document exactly what you accomplished, how and why you took the actions you did, and the impact your accomplishment had on the organization. Practice saying what you want to say and how you want to say it.

- **Implement the principles of proper speech.** Speak clearly, distinctly, and loudly enough to be heard by everyone in the room. This is especially important when communicating to groups. Avoid high-pitched tones. These are difficult to hear, especially for listeners who are middle-aged and older. Avoid what seems to be a bad habit for many speakers today: phrasing all communications as though they were questions.

- **Use appropriate body language.** Stand or sit erect. Maintain eye contact. Do not fidget or look away from your listeners. Do not cross your arms. When standing, your arms should be at your sides. When sitting, you may leave them in your lap or in a relaxed posture on the table or desk. It is always helpful to have your templates with documented evidence with you so that you can refer to them. However, do not shuffle papers while speaking. Do not tap your fingers or a pen on the desk or table as you speak. This is distracting. Practice presenting in front of a mirror so that you can critique your body language.

- **Be prepared for tough questions.** In staff development department meetings, practice delivering communication about evidence and have your colleagues question you about your findings. One of the most common questions is, "How can you be sure that it is education that made the difference?" Explain that you are not stating evidence as proof—you know that many variables contribute to successful outcomes. What you are saying is that before education, there was a certain problem, and after education the problem was reduced or resolved. That is the evidence you are presenting. You are not presenting it as "proof positive."

- **Start with your most impressive findings.** Begin with the results that show education has a positive impact on the organization. For example, if you have revised orientation according to evaluation data and input from staff nurses and nurse managers, you want to begin your presentation positively.

Communicate with confidence in writing

When communicating through writing, be concise and clear. Do not lead up to your results with a lot of excess information. Do not start out with a lengthy paragraph about reactive, learning, and behavioral data. Start with what will really capture attention: a concise statement about results. Many busy administrators will not read a complete report or entire committee minutes, so make sure the results that link education to a positive impact on the organization are identified in your very first sentence! For instance, your first statement might say something like, "Following the continuing education program on stroke rehabilitation, the average length of stay of stroke patients decreased by three days." This is an impressive result, and it offers evidence of the impact of education.

Suppose that your organization is pursuing accreditation as a regional center for the rehabilitation of stroke patients. The length of stay for stroke patients at your organization is above the national average. There are many factors that influence this problem, and education is one means of helping to resolve it. You have implemented an extensive education series concerning pathophysiology of stroke, acute care interventions, rehabilitation interventions, and patient/family education strategies. Six months after completion of this series, you are asked to submit to administration a written report about the effects of education. Your report should begin with hard-hitting impact statements such as follows.

Six months after implementation of stroke education, analysis shows that:
- *The length of stay for stroke patients is now that of the national average*
- *Monetary savings as a result of decreased lengths of stay are approximately $10,000 per patient*
- *There has been a 12% increase in patient independence in ADLs as measured by the organization's ADL scale*
- *Follow-up outpatient visits indicate a 15% increase in patient compliance with medication, exercise, and dietary regimens*

Additional findings show:
- *Nursing staff demonstrate a 15% increase in posttest scores following education*
- *Nursing staff demonstrate a 15% increase in application of knowledge as evidenced by behaviors on the stroke units*

As a result of these findings, all new members of the stroke team will participate in this education upon hire or transfer to these units. A refresher course will be offered on an annual basis to keep skills and knowledge current. This course is a computer-based learning program designed to be accessed at the learner's convenience and to reduce time away from patient units. New advances in care of the stroke patient will be communicated via in-service and on-the-job training as necessary.

Note that the results with the most significance to administration are the first statements in the report. Length of stay (a concern prior to education) and monetary impact are the first two items, followed by data pertaining to patient treatment outcomes. A bulleted list is easy to read and has a hard-hitting visual impact.

Statements about increase in knowledge and appropriate behaviors are important, but not what administration is most interested in. Certainly, you should include all pertinent results, but be sure to give precedence to those that grab the reader's attention. Remember, administration is not interested in a lengthy description of how you planned the education or a detailed description of its content. You can always provide this if requested, but it is usually not necessary. Most administrators and managers want a concise report of the results and are not necessarily concerned with how you achieved them.

Finally, the statement notes how you plan to help maintain knowledge and skills in ways that are cost-effective and convenient. These are two points that will make administration, managers, and staff happy.

Use language that everyone will understand

Whether you are communicating in person or in writing, make sure that you use language your audience will understand. If you are talking to staff development colleagues, it may be perfectly appropriate to talk about the five levels of program evaluation discussed in Chapter 3 or Malcolm Knowles' principles of adult education. However, other colleagues such as administrators, physical therapists, or information technology (IT) specialists will not understand jargon particular to the fields of staff development and adult education. Therefore, you need to know your audience. With whom will you be communicating? What are their priorities?

Looking at the preceding example of education to improve stroke patient outcome, you know that it is appropriate to use terms regarding length of stay and ADLs since these are terms common to everyone in your audience.

You know how frustrating it can be when IT specialists use jargon particular to their field when all you want to know is how long it will take for your computer to be up and running! The same can be said of NPD specialists who go into unnecessary detail about the various levels of evaluation, how data were collected, etc., when all the audience wants to know is "What were the results of education?"

When writing an especially critical report, or preparing a presentation, ask a trusted colleague from outside the staff development department to listen to your presentation and/or read your report for clarity and understanding. Be open to constructive criticism!

Make sure everyone in the staff development department communicates using EBP as a foundation

It is important that everyone in the staff development department communicates using EBP as a foundation. They should communicate with each other following the same principles of good communication that are used with every other audience. This will save time and help everyone to focus on results.

For example, suppose the NPD specialist in charge of nursing orientation is giving a report about recent revisions to the program during the staff development departmental meeting. She/he should begin with the most important results first and not start off with long, convoluted comments about how difficult the transition was or the opposition she/he faced. Results should come first, such as "New nurse turnover has decreased by 15% since the revisions have been in place." She/he may also explain other results from other levels of evaluation, such as the percentage of nurses who rated the orientation experience as excellent. But the focus needs to be on evidence. This doesn't mean that colleagues cannot share their triumphs or frustrations, but these feelings should not be the focus of the report or of the departmental meeting.

By focusing on evidence, the meetings will be more organized and take less time than if participants go off on tangents without a logical way of presenting information. Even the sharing of frustrations should be evidence-based. For example, opposition from managers about a change in the way a program has traditionally been presented needs to be dealt with. It's okay to vent for a short period of time, but the focus should be on gathering evidence to support the reason for the change and how to communicate this to the managers.

Use EBP as a tool to help you communicate more efficiently.

Deal with opposition effectively

We must anticipate dealing with opposition. It is inevitable. Let's say you want to use a blended learning approach for an important education program. Some staff and managers will want only a classroom approach, while others will want only a distance learning approach. Always assume that there will be some opposition to what you say. This way you can be prepared to deal with it and be pleasantly surprised if it doesn't occur.

Suppose you have done a pilot study that compares blended learning, total distance learning, and total classroom learning as teaching methodologies. The results from these programs provide evidence as to why you are making the change. Using evidence as a reason for a change is the best way to deal with opposition because evidence is objective. You are less likely to get into heated arguments or disagreements if you are using evidence and results as your reasons for a certain action.

That said, don't overlook the possibility of compromise. Other managers and staff members may have evidence to back up their concerns. Listen to what others are saying and be open to collaboration on strategies to identify and implement the best way to provide education.

Don't be afraid to use evidence to support your point of view, but also don't become rigid. Just remember that any revisions must be made after careful consideration and data analysis to determine evidence for the proper actions to take.

 The Survival of Staff Development

Resolve conflicts and opposing points of view

One of the best ways to resolve conflicts and opposition is to be prepared for the tough questions. In staff development department meetings, practice delivering communication about evidence and have your colleagues question you about your findings. Make sure that the questions are challenging. Two of the most common questions are, "How can you be sure that it is education that made the difference?" and "How can you ignore the contributions others have made?" You can explain that you are not stating evidence as proof. You know that many variables contribute to successful outcomes. What you are saying is that before education, there was a certain problem, and after education the problem was reduced or resolved. That is the evidence you are presenting.

> **STAFF DEVELOPMENT ALERT!** Don't use the words "proof" or "proven" in your presentations. There is no way to conclusively "prove" that education alone was responsible for particular results. All you can do is present evidence as to what occurred before and after education.

You should also acknowledge the contributions of others who have helped to make the results positive. For instance (going back to the earlier example involving stroke patients), after commenting that, following education, the length of stay of stroke patients is now in line with the national average, you can conclude your presentation by acknowledging the contributions of all of the direct patient care providers who contributed to this success.

Don't allow opposition to escalate into a full-blown verbal disagreement. Remain calm at all times. Never raise your voice. Assume a body posture that is open and non-threatening. Sit down and have the person who is opposing you sit down also. Keep your arms at your sides. Maintain eye contact. Do not make fists or cross your arms across your chest—both of these actions can be perceived as argumentative or threatening. Reiterate that you want to work together for the best possible patient outcomes and acknowledge, again, the contributions of everyone who contributed to the desired outcomes.

Figure 4.5 is a template to help you focus on the best way to communicate EBP findings.

Figure 4.5

Communicating EBP findings

In-person communication

1. How have you prepared?

2. Have you practiced your presentation so that you are implementing the principles of good speech?

3. Have you observed your body language in front of a mirror?

4. Have you identified the statements that will begin your presentation?

5. Are you using language everyone can understand?

In-writing communication

1. Have you begun your report with your most impressive findings?

2. Are your statements concise and clear?

3. Have you avoided unnecessary detail?

4. Are you using terminology everyone can understand?

Using EBP as a foundation

1. Do all members of the department understand what is meant by using evidence-based practice (EBP) as a focus for discussions?

2. Is evidence the focus of all communications among department members?

3. Is evidence the focus of departmental meetings?

Dealing with opposition

1. Do you have evidence to back up your position?

2. Have you identified the areas where compromise or program revisions are appropriate?

3. Have you included the "opposers" in the data gathering process?

Dealing with conflict

1. Have you acknowledged the contributions of persons other than those involved in staff development?

2. Have you used the word "evidence" as opposed to the word "proof"?

3. Have you practiced dealing with opposing points of view?

Here is a summary of communication principles pertaining to EBP in staff development:

- Communicate with confidence.

- Be brief. Start with statements that will grab the listener's or reader's attention immediately. This means starting with results that link education to organizational effectiveness.

- Use language that your listener will understand. Do not go into complicated explanations of adult learning principles, for example, and do not use verbiage that is common to educators but not so common to management or administration.

- Make sure that everyone in the staff development department is communicating using EBP as a foundation. EBP should be the norm and not the exception.

- Be prepared for opposition. Other departments may not like to hear you talking about evidence that links education to positive outcomes. They may say that their actions are just as relevant. Remember, you are not trying to say that staff development is more important than other departments; you are simply showing a link between education and a positive impact. Explain that you are not explaining the evidence that you have determined following analysis of education services. You are not using the word "proof," nor are you saying education is the only factor in the positive outcome. You are stating evidence based on your analysis of education.

When preparing to communicate findings from a complex project, you may need some help focusing. Figure 4.6 is an example of a template used for reporting a more complex project that requires extensive time and resources to implement. Note that in the evaluation data column, results data are presented first. In some circumstances, such as a question from an administrator, you may only need to state information from the evaluation column unless a more detailed explanation is requested.

> **STAFF DEVELOPMENT ALERT!** Communicate your evidence in person and in writing as often as possible to promote your department and yourself! Be brief yet effective, proclaiming your results as the data that will make an impression!

Figure 4.6

Administrative report on staff development EBP

Program title	Needs assessment data	Implementation method(s) and rationale	Evaluation data
Pathophysiology of Spinal Cord Injury: How to Intervene for Maximum Patient Outcomes	Eighty percent of RNs working on spinal cord injury (SCI) unit requested update on this topic on annual needs assessment survey. Nurse managers of the neuro-rehabilitation units noted that they documented a need for increased knowledge and application of knowledge concerning pathophysiology of SCI on 55% of RN performance evaluations. Length of stay for SCI patients on these units was four to seven days longer than estimated in 60% of patients. *Special comments:* The SCI rehabilitation program is relatively new. It has existed for 18 months. Fifty percent of the RNs are new to this specialty.	The program consists of blended learning—a computer-based learning component and a skills demonstration component. *Rationale:* The decision for blended learning was based on a pilot study of two groups of RNs: • Group I's continuing education was presented entirely in the classroom setting. • Group II participated in computer-based learning for the didactic portion of the course and then attended a skills lab. Successful completion of posttests and skills demonstration were as follows: • Group I: 90% • Group II: 95% Minor adjustments were made to the program, including better opportunities for question and answer sessions.	Length of stay for SCI patients was as estimated upon admission to the SCI program for 98% of patients admitted following implementation of this education program. Two percent of patients had longer than estimated lengths of stay, compared to 60% prior to program implementation. This program was offered over a period of six months. Ninety percent of RNs working on the neuro-rehabilitation units attended this program. All participants successfully completed the posttest and skills demonstration lab. Direct observation of nurses who attended the program found that 90% applied new knowledge and skills in the work setting.

Source: This figure was adapted from Evidence-Based Staff Development: Strategies to Create, Measure, and Refine Your Program *(2007), by Adrianne E. Avillion, DEd, RN.*

Using EBP to help you keep your job

EBP focuses on your accomplishments as well as areas for improvement. A focus on EBP practice provides evidence that you and your department make a positive difference, communicates accomplishments in an objective manner with data to justify your conclusions, organizes communication so that it is concise and clear, and allows you to demonstrate how you have contributed to the achievement of organizational goals and objectives.

In other words, EBP is the best way to demonstrate your value to the organization. It is also the best way to make administration think about what life might be like if there were no staff development department!

References

Avillion, A.E. (2007). Evidence-Based Staff Development: Strategies to Create, Measure, and Refine Your Program. Marblehead, MA: HCPro.

Avillion, A.E. (2008). *A Practical Guide to Staff Development: Evidence-Based Tools and Techniques for Effective Education* (2nd ed.). Marblehead, MA: HCPro.

Knowles, M. (1988). *The Modern Practice of Adult Education: From Pedagogy to Andragogy.* Cambridge, MA: The Cambridge Book Company.

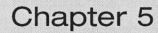

Chapter 5

Using Research to Solidify the Role of Staff Development

CHAPTER 5

Using Research to Solidify the Role of Staff Development

Introduction

Nursing research is an organized, systematic approach to solving and comprehending clinical problems. It is conducted to determine the effectiveness of specific nursing interventions and to provide evidence-based practice (EBP) for the nursing profession (Flaugher, 2008).

Nursing research activities are generally coordinated by nurse researchers, who are hired to be leaders in conducting research. They help nurses to identify research topics, write proposals, present proposals to investigational review boards, coordinate the research process, and present research findings (Flaugher, 2008). Although the position of nurse researcher is becoming more common, especially within teaching healthcare facilities, not all organizations have a nurse researcher on staff. Therefore, other options for acquiring the assistance of nursing research experts must be explored. Such options include collaborating with nurse researchers from other healthcare organizations, seeking guidance from professional associations, and/or working with individuals who offer their services as nurse researcher consultants.

How do you incorporate staff development into the research process in your own organization? How do you gain access to experts to help you conduct staff development research? The answers to these questions will not only help you to initiate staff development research but will also help you to enhance the security of your job and the staff development department.

What Is Staff Development Research?

Staff development research may be defined as an organized, systematic approach to identifying and resolving problems related to staff development practice. It is conducted to assess the effectiveness of education interventions, to provide EBP for the specialty of staff development, and to add to the unique body of knowledge that is staff development.

How does staff development research help solidify both the staff development department and individual staff development practitioners? Research is about having a positive impact on future practice that is based on scientific evidence. Research should foster a culture of staff development excellence. Such excellence should, in turn, translate into measurable evidence of staff development's impact on the organization.

Research findings provide evidence of what does and does not work in staff development. Staff development research is closely linked to clinical research since the focus of research in education is to determine what education strategies improve job performance, which in turn improves patient outcomes.

For example, suppose a staff nurse approaches a nurse researcher with the question, "How does staff communication influence the behavior of disruptive patients and families in the emergency department [ED]?" This is a good way for staff development personnel to become involved in research that highlights both education and clinical outcomes. In collaboration with the nurse researcher and the

ED staff, current communication patterns can be observed and analyzed with regard to their impact on disruptive patients and families. An education program can be developed and implemented based on this analysis. Following education of ED staff, communication patterns can be again observed and analyzed using the same methods as before. Ideally, communication will be enhanced and disruptive behaviors and their negative consequences diminished. Also ideally, the communication program can be offered to other departments, and its impact can be analyzed to determine whether communication can be improved throughout the organization.

The point is that collaboration among staff development, researchers, and clinical staff can help to improve job performance and patient outcomes. This kind of endeavor enhances the culture of staff development in several ways, the most obvious being that of improving the organization's effectiveness. But research also implies a sophistication of practice. Using research findings to enhance practice fosters enthusiasm not only for the research process but for actively pursuing excellence at advanced levels of practice.

What kinds of research questions can you think of that are appropriate for staff development collaboration? Here are some ideas to get you started:

- How does the education and training of preceptors influence retention of newly hired nurses?

- Does the establishment of a mentor program contribute to increased job satisfaction?

- How does distance learning compare to classroom-style learning for specific education topics?

- How does blended learning compare to all-classroom or all-distance learning in terms of learning, behavior, and results?

- Do mock emergency drills (e.g. cardiac arrest, bomb threats) have an impact on staff behaviors in the actual work setting?

- How does nursing orientation influence nursing retention?

Now, think about some research topic ideas that are purely concerned with staff development. Here are some ideas:

- How do staff development competencies influence job performance?

- Does the experience level of staff development personnel make a difference in the results of an education program?

- Does the education level of staff development personnel make a difference in the results of an education program?

- Does level of expertise correlate with burnout of staff development personnel?

- Does learner satisfaction with method of teaching impact learning, behavior, and results?

- Does learner satisfaction with faculty impact learning, behavior, and results?

- Does presentation of evidence as it relates to the impact of education have a positive effect on how other departments perceive staff development?

- Does presentation of evidence as it relates to the impact of education have a positive effect on the value administration places on staff development?

These are just some ideas of how research can be used in staff development. By using the findings from research projects such as these, you can improve staff development services and enhance your pursuit of staff development excellence.

Conducting Staff Development Research

Acquiring the help of experts

Most nursing professional development (NPD) specialists are not research experts, although they may have participated in various research projects. Gathering data pertaining to results is an excellent first step in the research process, but we still need to seek the help of experts when conducting formal research investigations. Here are some suggestions for acquiring help:

- **Contact the nurse researcher(s) in your organization.** If you are fortunate enough to have nurse researchers on staff, develop collaborative relationships with them. They are an invaluable resource! You may want to begin by sharing some of the evidence you have acquired that links staff development activities with changes/improvements in job performance or patient outcomes. You should also be prepared to share pertinent questions you have about your staff development practice that lend themselves to research (more later in the "Steps in the research process" section). The point is to come prepared to discuss research ideas. This holds true for any researcher you collaborate with, whether that researcher works within or outside of your organization.

- **Contact nurse researchers from other organizations.** With the approval of your administration, you may be able to collaborate with researchers from other organizations if your own facility does not have a nurse researcher. This type of collaboration is easier if you already have a professional rapport with staff development personnel from organizations that have nurse researchers on staff. A staff development research project that includes collaboration with multiple facilities can be an exciting endeavor!

> **STAFF DEVELOPMENT ALERT!** Before collaborating with researchers or any colleagues from organizations other than your own, be sure to obtain approval from your manager and/or administration. There may be political differences of which you are unaware that prohibit collaboration.

- **Investigate collaboration possibilities with colleges and universities.** Contact the departments of nursing at respected colleges and universities, particularly those with graduate programs. These programs will most likely have faculty with the necessary research expertise. Start by contacting those schools of nursing with which your organization has clinical affiliations.

- **Communicate with members of your professional associations on both the local and national level.** Professional associations such as the National Nursing Staff Development Organization *(www.nnsdo.org)* often offer research grants, collaboration possibilities, and a resource list of members who have expertise in various fields. The Honor Society of Nursing, Sigma Theta Tau International *(www.nursingsociety.org)*, is also an excellent resource when searching for help with research projects. Local chapters are affiliated with colleges and universities, and members are usually eager to assist their colleagues with research endeavors.

Accessing best practice data

Research projects generally involve accessing available best practice data from within and outside of your organization. Sources of these kinds of data include:

- Your own evidence of best practices identified from evaluation of your staff development products and services. Results data are especially helpful when identifying best practices.

- Review of staff development literature. A thorough literature is essential to any research project. Best practice data can be identified from the literature. Consult reliable journals such as *The Journal for Nurses in Staff Development* and *The Journal of Continuing Education in Nursing*. Professional associations and books that focus on staff development are other good sources of best practices.

> **STAFF DEVELOPMENT ALERT!** Just because information is published does not necessarily mean it is valid and/or reliable. Suggestions for conducting a literature review are presented later in this chapter.

- Best practices identified by professional associations. Professional associations often have a database of best practices. Associations also provide opportunities to network with colleagues who can provide best practice information.

As you work with your colleagues who are research experts, do not forget to ask them for suggestions about accessing best practice data. They may not be experts in staff development, but they *are* experts in knowing how to access a variety of online databases that may be helpful!

Using research findings to solidify the role of staff development

Research topics selected should reflect the goals of the organization. For example, you may be really interested in investigating the impact of orientation on retention. But if retention is good and administration has identified specific areas for improvement, such as decreasing the number of nosocomial infections, you would be wise to focus on organizational priorities.

Research should also be part of shared governance. Staff members as well as managers are now responsible (especially in ANCC Magnet Recognition® certified organizations) for the way patient care is delivered as well as patient outcomes. You may want to investigate how shared governance pertaining to education impacts specific patient outcomes. In a shared governance system, there is usually an education council, which helps to identify education needs, facilitates implementation of education, and collaborates on the analysis of findings to demonstrate results. Don't overlook shared governance councils as a source of research collaboration.

When analyzing research findings, think about how they correlate with administrative priorities. If research findings help to demonstrate staff development value, this can solidify your role within the organization.

Here are some questions to ask yourself when thinking about research as a means of solidifying the role of staff development:

- Have I made myself familiar with organizational priorities?

- Have I discussed how these priorities can be used in staff development research?

- Have I talked to my manager about how to correlate organizational priorities and staff development research?

- Have I collaborated with the nurse researcher(s) to choose projects that reflect organizational priorities?

- Have I gathered data from pertinent councils (e.g. education, quality improvement) to support my research ideas?

- Have I decided how research topics of interest to me will help to foster a culture of staff development excellence?

- Have I determined how research topics of interest to me will help to demonstrate the value of staff development to the organization?

- Have I objectively identified research topics that are of value to the organization, or have I overlooked such topics in preference to my own interests?

Staff development research will help us to identify strategies that will improve the way we deliver education. Improvements such as these should also help to improve results, those all-important links between education and organizational effectiveness. Make sure to include research projects and their results in your reports to management and administration. You need to keep them informed of the research you are conducting, the findings from that research, and how you plan to use those findings to improve your services. Research projects must be approved by your organization's institutional review board (IRB), which will require periodic updates as to your progress. But you need to think about how you will report your findings at the conclusion of your project as well.

For example, the template in Figure 4.6 in Chapter 4 is a good way to report your findings. When thinking about how to report findings, you need to address the following questions:

- With whom should I collaborate when writing the report? Who was instrumental in conducting this research project? The nurse researcher? Specific staff nurses? Managers? Physicians?

- Who should receive copies of this report? My manager? My colleagues? Administration?

- Has the report been written in an objective manner? Have I used words such as "findings" or "evidence" as opposed to "proven" or "proof"?

- Does the report indicate a need for further research? How will this research be conducted?

- Does the report include information pertaining to return on investment? Have I kept track of any expenses incurred as a result of the research?

- Does the report include information about how the research findings will be used to improve patient care? Job performance? Staff development practice?

- Does the report indicate possibilities for future collaborative research projects?

- Does the report indicate how future research may positively impact the organization?

Also remember that research projects make for excellent publication and presentation topics. As mentioned earlier, do not miss opportunities to publish or present your staff development accomplishments.

Publishing and/or presenting findings at conferences or conventions requires you to be prepared to discuss your research, but it also requires you to consider the political ramifications. For example, when preparing to present or publish, have you:

- Included the names of the key players in the project as coauthors? This can be a difficult dilemma. Suppose a physician was a major supporter of your project and helped to convince medical colleagues of its importance. This physician assisted in the research process, but in a minor way. Should the physician's name be included as an author in the published article? What are the consequences if the name is not included? Eliminating the physician's name from public credit may cause hard feelings and even cause this formerly supportive physician to oppose you in future endeavors. Politically, it is better to give key players acknowledgement whenever possible.

- Asked key players whether they want to be involved in publishing or presenting? Some may come right out with a negative response. Never include names of key persons without first getting their permission.

- Asked for assistance from experienced authors and/or presenters? If you do not have extensive publishing or presenting experience, don't be proud! Ask for help!

- Informed your manager and/or administration of your intent to publish or present? Usually, administration and management are pleased to have the organization presented in a positive manner. However, there may be factors of which you are unaware that make a public presentation of your research project unadvisable. Always check with management and administration before pursing publication or presentation.

Steps in the research process

The research process involves some very definite steps. A summary of the steps of the research process follows:

- **Select a topic:** What is it that interests you about staff development practice? You need to be interested in whatever research topic you choose. Research is not a quick and easy process. You need to have a passion for what you are investigating. What is it that bothers you about your practice? For instance, are you wondering why nurses are not transferring specific behaviors learned in the education setting to the work setting? How is orientation related to turnover? How does horizontal violence affect learning? What teaching method produces the best outcomes for a particular education topic? Work with your research expert to help narrow your focus and come up with a research question that is appropriate for investigation.

- **Perform a literature review:** A literature review is conducted to narrow the focus and identify information about best practices as well as to find out what other investigators have discovered about your research topic. Internet search engines are generally the primary sources of literature reviews. However, it is important to evaluate the quality of Internet sources. Figure 5.1 will help you to do this.

  Examples of some reliable search engines include:

  - Cumulative Index to Nursing and Allied Health Literature *(www.cinahl.com)*

  - EBSCOhost *(www.ebsco.com)*

  - MEDLINE *(www.nimh.nih.gov)*

  - PubMed *(www.pubmed.gov)*

- **Select a research design:** The design includes selecting the setting, participants or subjects, the time period of the research, cost, interventions (e.g., teaching method), tools or instruments to be used to collect data, how the data is to be analyzed, and how findings will be communicated. Ethics are also part of the research design. As your research design is developed, you must be sure that all investigators conduct the research honestly and without bias, that human rights are not violated, and that the research will not cause participants physical or psychological harm.

- **Presentation to the IRB:** IRB committees are responsible for ensuring that participants' rights and welfare are protected while the study is conducted (Flaugher, 2008). You must follow your organization's policy for research and IRB review.

 The Survival of Staff Development

- **Implementation of research design:** After receiving IRB approval, you will implement your research design. In conjunction with your research expert, you will then critique your findings and describe your conclusions.

- **Communicate your findings:** Communicate your findings to appropriate persons within your organization. Explain how you will use those findings to improve staff development services. Use your research project as a basis for a journal article or presentation at an education conference.

Figure 5.1

Evaluation of Internet sources

1. Who is the author? Are the author's credentials listed? Is there an e-mail address or a way of contacting the author if questions arise? Is the researcher the person who is responsible for the creation of the site?

2. When determining accuracy, are references listed? Does the article seem credible? Is the article based on information that the reader already knows to be true? Is statistical data listed, and if so, is it presented in graphs or tables for clear understanding?

3. Is the document current? When was the site created? Is there any indication that the information is updated or revised frequently? Are there links to other websites? Are these links current?

4. Is the site free of advertising? If advertising is present, is it separated from the written material? Is the information objective and free from author bias? Does it include provocative language? What is the URL of the document? Does it reside on the Web server of an organization that may have extreme points of view?

5. Does the site appear to be complete, or are there references to additional sources that complete the information presented?

6. What is the main purpose of the site? Is its emphasis technical, scholarly, popular, or other?

7. Is the site easy to use, or is special software required? If the latter is true, can the software be downloaded free of cost? Is the site open to anyone with access to the Internet?

In summary, staff development research is important to the survival of your department and to the survival of the specialty. Without research, there is little chance to determine best practices and benchmarks for the profession. How do research findings contribute to departmental and specialty survival?

- Research findings of best practices and benchmarks add to the unique body of knowledge that is staff development

- The research process helps to nurture proficient and expert NPD specialists by providing new opportunities to contribute to the organization

- The research process offers opportunities for individual recognition of accomplishments

- Research findings demonstrate staff development impact on job performance and patient outcomes

- Research findings guide staff development practice by showing strengths and weaknesses of current practice and suggested revisions for the future

Findings should be used not only to improve your own practice but to add to the unique body of knowledge that is staff development. They can also be used to nurture NPD specialists and provide personal recognition!

Reference

Flaugher, M. (2008). *Nursing Research Program Builder: Strategies to Translate Findings into Practice.* Marblehead, MA: HCPro.

Chapter 6

Some Thoughts on Personal Survival

CHAPTER 6

Some Thoughts on Personal Survival

LEARNING OBJECTIVE

After reading this chapter, you will be able to:

- Identify personal survival skills

Introduction

Most healthcare professionals, particularly younger ones, no longer identify themselves by their workplace. We have seen mergers, downsizing, and budget cuts to extents not thought possible only a few decades ago. Professionally, we define ourselves by what we do, not where we work.

We have a responsibility to do our best for our organizations and for our departments. But we are primarily responsible to ourselves for our own professional growth and development. Individual survival is, arguably, our greatest challenge and our greatest responsibility. Healthcare professionals who are functioning at their maximum capabilities will not only enhance their personal survival, but will contribute to departmental survival by the excellence of their job performance.

Tips for Personal Survival

Trust your instincts

As mentioned in Chapter 1, trust your instincts. If you "feel" more than "see" a problem, do not discount your feelings—there are probably good reasons for them. Ask yourself:

- Has there been a change in the way your manager treats you?

- Has there been a change in the way the manager of staff development is being treated by her or his manager?

- Have there been changes, or rumored changes, in the organizational structure?

- Are other colleagues expressing thoughts of uneasiness about the organization's future?

- Have you been asked to decrease spending or to hold off on purchases that had already been approved?

- Have your colleagues from other organizations heard rumors that your organization is having problems (e.g., financial, accreditation)?

Instincts can often be backed up by objective evidence if you take the time to look for it. If your instincts are telling you that there is trouble ahead, believe them!

Look at how your department is conducting business

Your personal survival depends, in part, on how your department is conducting business. If you are part of a department that is not grounded in evidence-based practice (EBP), it is likely that the department will be vulnerable to budget and position cuts. EBP allows you (and your department) to provide evidence to administration, management, and other departments that shows how you influence patient outcomes and job performance.

Determine how your department is perceived by the rest of the organization. If others fail to see the department's value, it is likely that they will question your individual professional worth as well.

Here are some questions you must answer regarding how your department conducts its business:

- Is your department grounded in staff development EBP? If not, what can you do to encourage its implementation?

- Have you based your own practice on the concepts of EBP? Can you produce evidence that your job performance has a positive impact on the organization?

- Does your department stay within its budget? If not, why not? What can you do to help stay within budget?

- Do the members of your department support each other? Do you function as a team or are there significant internal conflicts? If conflicts exist, can they be resolved?

- What kind of reputation does your department have within the organization? Is your work respected, or do other departments have no idea what staff development does?

- How are the accomplishments of your department and of individual members of your department communicated to administration?

- Does your department have a business plan? If so, is it used as a guideline for departmental functioning? If your department does not have a business plan, can you promote the establishment of such a plan?

- Does your department gather data from all five levels of evaluation? If not, why not? If so, how are the data analyzed and used to improve staff development products and services?

Take a good, hard, objective look at the way your department conducts business. Staff development is a business and should be conducted as such.

Have a plan to deal with downsizing

Although downsizing is a common phenomenon, most people tend to think, "It can't happen to me." Unfortunately, it can happen to anyone and everyone. As part of your personal survival, you should:

- Have some money saved as an emergency fund in case of job loss.

- Keep abreast of job openings in your field in your geographic area if you cannot relocate and in preferred locations if you are able to relocate.

- Always keep your résumé up to date.

- Strive for personal accomplishments, such as publishing and presenting, that showcase your individual talents.

- Be alert to vacancies that are not filled in your organization. This may be a signal of job eliminations to come.

- Know your rights. Know how much sick time and vacation time you have accrued. Review your organization's policies on downsizing, layoffs, and terminations.

- Travel light. Downsizing, when it occurs, is often abrupt, leaving the affected person little time to gather and remove personal belongings.

- Maintain your professionalism. If you are faced with downsizing, never lose your temper, make accusations, or become verbally or physically aggressive.

- Don't vent your frustrations online. Never ever write comments about your downsizing or your former employer in e-mail, Twitter, Facebook, etc.

Pay attention to your own continuing education

Make sure you are up to date on the latest developments in your field. Pursue that graduate degree or certification that you have been planning to earn. Find a mentor. Identify your career goals and develop a plan for attaining them. It is imperative that you keep abreast of changes in the staff development and adult education field. Here are some suggestions for doing so:

- Pursue continuing education contact hours specific to the field of staff development. These types of contact hours are accessible online from the National Nursing Staff Development Organization (NNSDO), at conferences and conventions that focus on staff development, and at research-focused programs such as those offered by the Honor Society of Nursing (Sigma Theta Tau International: *www.nursingsociety.org*).

- Pursue formal academic graduate credits in adult education and/or research.

- Read publications pertaining to adult professional development and continuing education in fields other than healthcare. The American Society for Training & Development (ASTD) is a good example of an association that offers valuable information for adult educators regardless of their specialty or discipline.

- Read business-related publications such as *The Wall Street Journal* for economics and healthcare trends.

- Network with colleagues locally, nationally, and internationally. The Internet allows for global communication and networking with a click of the mouse.

Join professional associations

Be an active member of your professional associations. They are excellent sources for networking. Be willing to serve on committees and task forces. Share your expertise. Be willing to serve as a mentor. People who are willing to help others are more likely to receive help when they need it.

Here are some examples of professional associations that may be helpful to you:

- **NNSDO:** The NNSDO's vision is to "establish itself as the most influential authority and thought leadership body for nursing professional development, through focusing our efforts on data driven outcomes grounded by a comprehensive knowledge repository" (NNSDO, 2011). The NNSDO has an annual convention, online learning opportunities, and extensive publications devoted to the practice of staff development. There are excellent opportunities for networking as well. Membership benefits include the association's journal, *The Journal for Nurses in Staff Development*. Access the NNSDO website at *www.nnsdo.org*.

- **ASTD:** According to the organization, "ASTD is the world's largest association dedicated to workplace learning and performance professionals" (ASTD, 2011). The ASTD has members from more than 100 countries. The organization offers an extensive array of educational resources and networking opportunities. Access the ASTD website at *www.astd.org*.

- **American Association for Adult and Continuing Education (AAACE):** The AAACE is "dedicated to the belief that lifelong learning contributes to human fulfillment and positive social change. We envision a more humane world made possible by the diverse practice of our members in helping adults acquire the knowledge, skills and values needed to lead productive and satisfying lives" (AAACE, 2011). There are several publications associated with the organization, including *Adult Education Quarterly*. Networking and education are important components of this organization. Access the AAACE website at *www.aaace.org*.

Know when it is time to jump ship

Sometimes, your best career option is to seek employment elsewhere. This may be difficult for a variety of reasons. You may have spent many years with your current employer and have developed close friendships with colleagues. You may believe that the problems you face are surmountable. However, part of your survival skills must include deciding when your current position is simply untenable.

If you spend more work hours frustrated than satisfied, it may be time to leave. If you have proposed innovations that would make you (and your department) more secure, only to have those innovations ignored or belittled, it may be time to leave. If there are no opportunities to achieve your own career goals, it may be time to leave. If you spend more days unhappy with your career than happy, it may be time to leave. Have the courage to take an honest look at your career and make the decision that is best for you, no matter how challenging it may seem.

If you are happy with your career, use your knowledge and skills to grow professionally. Give your best efforts to your department and to your organization. Gather evidence that demonstrates your value to the organization as well as your department's value. Pursue research opportunities that help improve staff development services and add to the specialty's body of knowledge. And do not forget to enjoy the journey that is part of a career in staff development!

References

American Association for Adult and Continuing Education. (2011). What's happening at AAACE. Retrieved May 16, 2011, from *www.aaace.org.*

American Society for Training & Development. (2011). About us. Retrieved May 16, 2011, from *www.astd.org/ASTD/aboutus.*

National Nursing Staff Development Organization. (2011). NNSDO vision. Retrieved May 16, 2011, from *www.nnsdo.org.*

Nursing Education
Instructional Guide

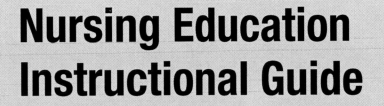

Target Audience

The target audiences of this book include staff development professionals, directors of staff development, nurse managers, charge nurses, chief nursing officers, chief nurse executives, directors of nursing, vice presidents of nursing, vice presidents of patient care services, nurse preceptors, and clinical nurse leaders.

Statement of Need

This book is a survival guide for staff development specialists and nursing development specialists. It covers orientation and critical thinking strategies for strengthening the staff development department into a department that has a measurable impact on the organization. The book features practical examples and tools and can be used by staff development professionals to increase their competence and demonstrate the value of their department. (This activity is intended for individual use only.)

Educational Objectives

Upon completion of this activity, participants should be able to:

- Identify the characteristics of a survivor mentality

- Explain how to focus on evidence when analyzing staff development products and services

- Design a staff development departmental structure that facilitates the design and implementation of products and services

- Identify components of a staff development business plan

- Align the components of a staff development business plan with organizational goals and objectives

- Correlate the components of a staff development business plan with evidence-based practice (EBP) in staff development

- Explain the concept of EBP in staff development

- Correlate EBP in staff development to departmental and job survival

- Perform all levels of program evaluation from the perspective of EBP in staff development

- Link EBP to specific staff development products and services

- Identify specific outcomes per EBP in staff development

- Communicate EBP in staff development findings effectively

- Explain why staff development research is important to the staff development department, to individual departments, and to individual practitioners

- Discuss steps in the research process

- Explain how to use research findings to solidify the role of staff development

- Identify personal survivor skills

Faculty

Adrianne E. Avillion, DEd, RN, is the owner of Avillion's Curriculum Design in York, PA. She specializes in designing continuing education programs for healthcare professionals and freelance medical writing. She also offers consulting services in work redesign, quality improvement, and staff development.

Continuing Education

Nursing Contact Hours

HCPro, Inc., is accredited as a provider of continuing nursing education by the American Nurses Credentialing Center Commission on Accreditation.

This educational activity for 2 nursing contact hours is provided by HCPro, Inc.

Faculty Disclosure Statement

HCPro, Inc., has confirmed that none of the faculty, contributors, or planners have any relevant financial relationships to disclose related to the content of this educational activity.

Disclosure of Unlabeled Use

This educational activity may contain discussion of published and/or investigational uses of agents that are not indicated by the FDA. HCPro, Inc., does not recommend the use of any agent outside of the labeled indications. The opinions expressed in the educational activity are those of the faculty and do not necessarily represent the views of HCPro, Inc. Please refer to the official prescribing information for each product for discussion of approved indications, contraindications, and warnings.

Instructions

In order to be eligible to receive your nursing contact hours for this activity, you are required to do the following:

1. Read the book *The Survival of Staff Development*

2. Complete the exam and receive a passing score of 80% or higher

3. Complete the evaluation

4. Provide your contact information on the exam and evaluation

5. Submit exam and evaluation to HCPro, Inc.

Please provide all of the information requested above and mail or fax your completed exam, program evaluation, and contact information to:

> HCPro, Inc.
> Attention: Continuing Education Manager
> 75 Sylvan Street, Suite A-101
> Danvers, MA 01923
> Fax: 781/639-7857

NOTE

This book and associated exam are intended for individual use only. If you would like to provide this continuing education exam to other members of your nursing or physician staff, please contact our customer service department at 877/727-1728 to place your order. The exam fee schedule is as follows:

Exam Quantity	Fee
1	$0
2–25	$15 per person
26–50	$12 per person
51–100	$8 per person
101+	$5 per person

Continuing Education Exam

Name: _____

Title: _____

Facility name: _____

Address: _____

Address: _____

City: _____ State: _____ ZIP: _____

Phone number: _____ Fax number: _____

E-mail: _____

Date completed: _____

1. Which of the following statements pertaining to a survivor mentality is correct?

    a. Survivors avoid asking management and administration questions that are challenging

    b. Survivors gather evidence pertaining to all staff development products and services

    c. Survivors pursue continuing education exclusively in the field of staff development

    d. Survivors trust objective data and should not be misled by their instincts

2. A focus on evidence requires which of the following?

    a. The essence of EBP in staff development must show evidence of a link between education, job performance, and patient outcomes

    b. All staff development products and services must be analyzed simultaneously

    c. EBP in staff development is primarily the responsibility of the manager of the staff development department

    d. EBP identification is not possible for programs such as improving communication skills

3. Which of the following reflects a departmental structure that enhances survivorship?

   a. A staff development department that has the same job descriptions for unit-based educators and nursing professional development (NPD) specialists

   b. A vice president position in staff development that requires preparation at the baccalaureate level

   c. A staff development department that makes a distinction between competent and proficient NPD specialists

   d. A managerial position in staff development that reports to a nurse manager

4. "X Community Hospital advocates lifelong learning for all of its employees." This type of statement is most likely part of a _____ statement.

   a. mission

   b. vision

   c. values

   d. description

5. A realistic, future-oriented statement is a:

   a. Philosophy

   b. Vision statement

   c. Values statement

   d. Mission statement

6. Which of the following is a best practice concerning departmental structure and function?

   a. Identify by name who holds each position in the department

   b. Include an organizational chart for the department

   c. Provide detailed descriptions of the committees that personnel attend

   d. Avoid identifying partnerships because this may cause a conflict of interest with competing organizations

7. Which of the following is an appropriate objective on an action plan?

    a. Improve Advanced Cardiac Life Support (ACLS) certification passing rate among critical care nurses

    b. Increase link between education and reduction in medical errors

    c. Implement initiatives to reduce medication errors

    d. Design and implement a distance learning course on pathophysiology of pancreatic cancer by the end of this fiscal year

8. EBP in staff development:

    a. Relies on behavioral evidence as the data that demonstrates education's impact on the organization

    b. Helps to close the gap between identified best practices and actual staff development practice

    c. Requires that return on investment (ROI) be calculated on all staff development products and services

    d. Does not need to incorporate reaction and learning data

9. Which of the following statements pertaining to EBP in staff development and job/departmental survival is accurate?

    a. Implementation of EBP in staff development guarantees job security

    b. EBP is primarily the responsibility of the manager of the staff development department

    c. EBP in staff development is linked to committee and council activities as well as education programs

    d. Implementation of EBP in staff development does not include using publications and presentations created by staff development personnel

10. Following demonstration of a new piece of equipment, learners are required to demonstrate competency in a skills laboratory setting in a classroom environment. This is an example of:

    a. Learning

    b. Behavior

    c. Results

    d. ROI

11. Following implementation of a program on infection control initiatives, the rate of nosocomial infections decreases by 15%. This is an example of:

    a. Learning

    b. ROI

    c. Behavior

    d. Results

12. An instructor who teaches ACLS is given high praise on participant evaluations. This is an example of:

    a. Reaction

    b. Learning

    c. Behavior

    d. Results

13. When analyzing your orientation program:

    a. You can eliminate gathering reaction data if you have limited time and resources

    b. Analyze data from each level of evaluation in isolation

    c. Be sure to incorporate turnover data as part of your analysis

    d. Avoid linking retention data to specific preceptors

14. When communicating staff development evidence:

    a. Report evidence during committees only when specifically asked to do so

    b. Begin by presenting your reactive data findings

    c. Avoid bringing completed templates with you

    d. Anticipate tough questions and practice how you will respond to them

15. Which of the following statements about communicating EBP is correct?

    a. Publications have little or no impact in EBP communication

    b. Results data should be presented first

    c. In-service education evaluations yield little results data as they are often presented as on-the-job training efforts

    d. Continuing education programs are the primary sources of EBP data

16. Which of the following statements pertaining to staff development research is accurate?

    a. Nursing staff development research activities are generally coordinated by physicians

    b. Staff development research is conducted to assess the effectiveness of education interventions

    c. Nurse researchers must also be experts in staff development in order to facilitate staff development research

    d. Research activities should be confined to your own organization

17. You can use staff development research to enhance departmental survival by:

    a. Using the results to hire a staff development nurse researcher

    b. Using the findings to improve services

    c. Sharing the findings with administration only if the research results are positive

    d. Sharing the findings with nurse researchers from other organizations

18. When conducting research, it is important to:

    a. Rely on Internet sources because they can be assumed to be reliable

    b. Select a topic that is of primary interest to your manager

    c. Select best practices from sources other than your own results

    d. Determine how you will communicate findings as part of your research design

Continuing Education Exam Answer Key

(Please record all exam and evaluation answers here)

Name: _____ License #: _____

Facility: _____ Title: _____

Address: _____

City: _____ State: _____ ZIP: _____

Phone: _____ E-mail: _____

(Certificates are e-mailed to learners unless otherwise stated here)

Please record the letter of the correct answer to the corresponding exam question below:					
1.	2.	3.	4.	5.	6.
7.	8.	9.	10.	11.	12.
13.	14.	15.	16.	17.	18.

Continuing Education Evaluation

1 = Strongly agree	2 = Agree	3 = Disagree	4 = Strongly disagree

(Please rate the responses below according to the scale above to rate the quality of this educational activity.)

1. Please indicate how well you feel this activity met the learning objectives listed: 1   2   3   4

2. Objectives were related to the overall purpose/goal of the activity: 1   2   3   4

3. This activity was related to my continuing education needs: 1   2   3   4

4. The exam for the activity was an accurate test of the knowledge gained: 1   2   3   4

5. The activity avoided commercial bias or influence: 1   2   3   4

6. This activity met my expectations: 1   2   3   4

7. The format was an appropriate method for delivery of the content for this activity: 1   2   3   4

8. Will this activity enhance your professional practice?   Yes   No

9. How much time did it take for you to complete this activity? _____

10. Do you have any additional comments on this activity? _____

_____

Return completed form to:

HCPro, Inc. • Attention: Continuing Education Manager • 75 Sylvan Street, Suite A-101, Danvers, MA 01923 • Tel 877/727-1728 • Fax 781/639-7857

© 2011 HCPro, Inc.   **The Survival of Staff Development**